Cultures of Femininity in Modern Fashion

Cultures of Femininity in Modern Fashion

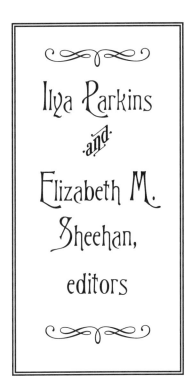

Ilya Parkins

·and·

Elizabeth M. Sheehan,

editors

UNIVERSITY OF NEW HAMPSHIRE PRESS
DURHAM, NEW HAMPSHIRE

UNIVERSITY OF NEW HAMPSHIRE PRESS
An imprint of University Press of New England
www.upne.com
© 2011 University of New Hampshire
Manufactured in the United States of America
Designed by Kathrine Kimball
Typeset in Bembo by Integrated Publishing Solutions

For permission to reproduce any of the material in this book, contact Permissions,
University Press of New England, One Court Street, Suite 250, Lebanon NH 03766;
or visit www.upne.com

Library of Congress Cataloging-in-Publication Data appear
on the last printed page of this book.

5 4 3 2 1

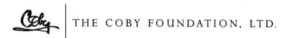 THE COBY FOUNDATION, LTD.

The editors and publisher gratefully acknowledge the support of the
Coby Foundation, Ltd.

Becoming Modern: New Nineteenth-Century Studies

SERIES EDITORS

Sarah Way Sherman
Department of English
University of New Hampshire

Rohan McWilliam
Anglia Ruskin University
Cambridge, England

Janet Aikins Yount
Department of English
University of New Hampshire

Janet Polasky
Department of History
University of New Hampshire

This book series maps the complexity of historical change and assesses the formation of ideas, movements, and institutions crucial to our own time by publishing books that examine the emergence of modernity in North America and Europe. Set primarily but not exclusively in the nineteenth century, the series shifts attention from modernity's twentieth-century forms to its earlier moments of uncertain and often disputed construction. Seeking books of interest to scholars on both sides of the Atlantic, it thereby encourages the expansion of nineteenth-century studies and the exploration of more global patterns of development.

For a complete list of books available in this series, see www.upne.com

Ilya Parkins and Elizabeth M. Sheehan, editors, *Cultures of Femininity in Modern Fashion*

Brian Joseph Martin, *Napoleonic Friendship: Military Fraternity, Intimacy, and Sexuality in Nineteenth-Century France*

Andrew Taylor, *Thinking America: New England Intellectuals and the Varieties of American Identity*

Elizabeth A. Fay, *Fashioning Faces: The Portraitive Mode in British Romanticism*

Katherine Joslin, *Edith Wharton and the Making of Fashion*

Daneen Wardrop, *Emily Dickinson and the Labor of Clothing*

Ronald D. LeBlanc, *Slavic Sins of the Flesh: Food, Sex, and Carnal Appetite in Nineteenth-Century Russian Fiction*

Barbara Penner, *Newlyweds on Tour: Honeymooning in Nineteenth-Century America*

Christine Levecq, *Slavery and Sentiment: The Politics of Feeling in Black Atlantic Antislavery Writing, 1770–1850*

Jennifer J. Popiel, *Rousseau's Daughters: Domesticity, Education, and Autonomy in Modern France*

Paula Young Lee, editor, *Meat, Modernity, and the Rise of the Slaughterhouse*

Duncan Faherty, *Remodeling the Nation: The Architecture of American Identity, 1776–1858*

Jennifer Hall-Witt, *Fashionable Acts: Opera and Elite Culture in London, 1780–1880*

Reading Dress Series

SERIES EDITORS

Katherine Joslin
Department of English
Western Michigan University

Daneen Wardrop
Department of English
Western Michigan University

This series engages questions about clothing, textiles, design, and production in relation to history, culture, and literature in its many forms. Set primarily in the long nineteenth century, it examines the emergence of modernity by exploring the interweaving of material culture with social history and literary texts in ways that resonate with readers and scholars at the turn into the twenty-first century. The editors seek books that offer fresh ways of relating fashion to discourse and of understanding dress in the context of social, cultural, and political history. Such topics might include, for example, analyzing American, British, and/or European notions of style or tracing the influence of developing modes of production. As with the Becoming Modern series generally, the editors especially welcome books with transatlantic focus or that appeal to a transatlantic audience.

Reading Dress is a subseries of Becoming Modern: New Nineteenth–Century Studies published by the University Press of New Hampshire.

Ilya Parkins and Elizabeth M. Sheehan, editors, *Cultures of Femininity in Modern Fashion*
Katherine Joslin, *Edith Wharton and the Making of Fashion*
Daneen Wardrop, *Emily Dickinson and the Labor of Clothing*

To the memory of Barbara Godard
—ILYA PARKINS

To Beth, Bob, and Chris
—ELIZABETH SHEEHAN

Contents

III. Fashion and the Materiality of Gender

Acknowledgments

The editors are grateful to Paul Fortunato for inspiring their collaboration on this collection. We also thank Richard Pult of University Press of New England for his good humor, patience, and wisdom. We are indebted to the University of British Columbia Okanagan's Internal Grants program. Elizabeth Sheehan gratefully acknowledges the support of the University of Virginia and, in particular, of Professor Deborah E. McDowell.

Permission granted to publish a revised version of Ellen Rosenman's essay, "Fear of Fashion; or, How the Coquette Got Her Bad Name." The original appeared in ANQ 15, no. 3 (2002): 12–21. Published by Heldref Publications, 1319 Eighteenth St., NW, Washington, DC 20036-1802. Copyright ©2002.

The authors gratefully acknowledge the generous support of the Coby Foundation, Ltd.

Ilya Parkins and
Elizabeth M. Sheehan

INTRODUCTION

Cultures of Femininity in Modern Fashion

In a concluding commentary on a 2008 essay collection on the figuration of the Modern Girl in the early twentieth century, historian Kathy Peiss asserts that "much of the literature on the Modern Girl in the United States [. . .] tends to separate leisure, consumption, and marketing from the domain of formal politics."[1] Peiss's observation indicates an ideological partition of leisure and consumption from political and economic life. This distinction feminizes, and hence trivializes and dismisses, consumption as a force in the consolidation of the modern, thereby continually writing the history of modernity as a masculine project.

Like Peiss and the authors of *The Modern Girl Around the World*, other recent scholars have challenged long-standing associations between modernity and masculinity to show how images and ideas of femininity shaped concepts of "the modern." For instance, scholars have complicated classic accounts of modernity, such as Marshall Berman's *All That Is Solid Melts into Air*, which establishes a masculine individual as the paradigmatic subject of modernity.[2] Work on consumer culture in particular has been pivotal to countering the many accounts of modernity that present women as anterior to or excluded from it. Sartorial fashion has at times figured in such work (including the *Modern Girl* collection), often as an example of how the image of modern women featured in visual culture or as evidence of the growing reach of commodity culture in the late nineteenth and early twentieth centuries. Yet fashion has received little attention as a gendered phenomenon that not only reflected but also influenced how modernity and femininity were conceived and experienced. As *Cultures of Femininity in Modern Fashion* shows, fashion was pivotal to how "ordinary women," artists, writers, and social critics understood and articulated what it meant to be modern. Moreover, fashion offers an important means to expand our understanding of the relationship between femininity and modernity by allowing us to draw connections between women as symbols or objects *and* women as agents of the modern. That is, fashion links gendered representations of the modern to women's experiences of modernity and thus helps us to see how women navigated their position as modern subjects. In doing so, fashion enables us to conceptualize modernity not as an imposition, but rather as a negotiation. In turn, if we understand modernity as a negotiation, accomplished (in part) through fashion, we can begin to bridge persistent divides not only between subject and object, but also between consumption and politics, self and society, the symbolic and the material, and the everyday and the monumental, which persist in discussions of modernity.

In this introduction we lay out the ways in which fashion offers a feminist intervention in discussions of modernity. But before we outline these areas of intervention, we must spend a few moments defining our terms. What do we mean by modernity, by fashion, and by femininity? With regard to modernity, we work indebted to those scholars who have crafted a cultural approach to this concept, one that attends to the multiple scenes of transformation that occurred in most of the West and many other parts of the world in the nineteenth and early twentieth centuries. This includes what is usually glossed as modernization by social scientists: industrialization, urbanization, the introduction of new technologies and practices that reworked everyday experiences of time and place, in locales ranging from the city street to the workplace. It includes the political and ideological horizon, in which a concept of liberal individualism and democratic ideals came to govern the lives of Western subjects, and in which the self reigned supreme, giving rise to a collective project, a labor, of selfhood.[3] Finally, it includes the aesthetic dimension that became visible in the latter half of the nineteenth century: works of art and of literature that responded to new realms of experience opened by technological and ideological transformations, often by pushing at the limits of form through self-conscious experimentation with aesthetic and social convention. The new modernist studies that has flourished in the last decade recognizes these multiple scenes of modernity as interlocking and mutually constitutive, and in doing so often straddles the boundary between humanities and social scientific inquiry. This is also a field in which a pervasive top-down model—one that conceived of modernity as a Western, metropolitan invention imposed upon rural or colonial subjects and upon women, who were essentially located outside modernity—has given way to the more nuanced understanding that, in

Dilip Gaonkar's words, "people 'make' themselves modern, as opposed to being 'made' modern by alien and impersonal forces."[4] This is the field of modernist studies as it is currently configured, and as this collection shows, an interdisciplinary, cultural approach is well suited to the particular character of fashion—a fact that makes it all the more timely to introduce a feminist analysis of fashion to this field and to scholarship that describes the contours and meaning of modernity in art, culture, and politics.

"Fashion" refers most simply to ongoing stylistic change in dress. Understood in these terms, fashion is intertwined with many of the changes that have come to define modernity—from the rise of mass production and consumption to the proliferation of popular media and visual culture. The connection between fashion and modernity has, in fact, been long established; key theorists of modernity, including Georg Simmel and Walter Benjamin, identified fashion as exemplary of the modern.[5] To Simmel, fashion demonstrated the tension between the desires for individuation and assimilation that characterized modern democracy. For Benjamin, fashion epitomized the modern bourgeois thirst for the new, which was paradoxically also a desire to remake the past in its own image, just as dress styles adapt older modes to suit new purposes. Decades before Simmel and Benjamin, Charles Baudelaire linked fashion to modern aesthetics, as he famously identified *la mode* as an ideal subject through which to capture *modernité*, defined as "the transient, the fleeting, the contingent; it is one half of art, the other being the eternal and the immovable."[6] More recent critics—including Elizabeth Wilson, Ulrich Lehmann, and Caroline Evans—have drawn upon the work of these nineteenth- and early twentieth-century critics to articulate the relationship between fashion and modernity.[7] In her important study, *Adorned in Dreams: Fashion and Modernity*, Wilson defines fashion and modernity by their mutual emphasis on constant change, and she also analyzes fashion as central to the fragmented, processual nature of modern selfhood.

We take femininity to consist of a constellation of significations, which is enacted through a broad range of behaviors, practices, and affects, and thereby becomes naturalized as belonging to female-bodied people. Femininity can be understood as ideological in the purest sense; the meanings and practices associated with it are so pervasive that they gain the status of social truth and, importantly, are seen as residing in the biology of female-bodied people (just as masculinity, as a dichotomously premised category, is generally understood as an effect of male biology). The definition of femininity that guides us thus stresses its *material* reproduction through the bodies of subjects and—as this volume foregrounds—in the relations among subjects, and between subjects and institutions. Femininity is an embodied orientation as much as it is a discursive construct; it is sustained as a social category, as Judith Butler's work has allowed us to see, through its repetitive iteration in individual bodily comportment and practices.[8] A range of social theorists of gender also have also made it clear that femininity possesses such normative strength that it is often enforced in coercive or even violent ways upon the self and others.

In taking up a definition of femininity, we contend that there are a number of ways in which fashion can help us "see" femininity more clearly, adding depth to our understanding of this gender category. Femininity can certainly be disarticulated from female-bodied people (which helps to construct our understandings of the "female body" as such) and can be disarticulated from subjects altogether, as fashion shows. Indeed, fashion is an excellent example of a feminized material object, which both takes on and helps to produce the material practices of femininity. Thus, when in this volume we refer to cultures of femininity, we include fashion as a feminine actor, a vector of the kinds of significations and practices that help to constitute femininity as an ideological construct. But, as a number of essays suggest, fashion can also be seen as materially challenging regimes of gender in modernity; Elizabeth Sheehan and Lori Harrison-Kahan, for instance, investigate the ways that fashion could disrupt naturalized racial, ethnic and gender politics, and Jasmine Rault suggests that it functioned as a dissembling agent, one that helped constitute a community of women who lived their gender and sexuality in oppositional ways.

In addition, femininity has historically been posited in a binary relationship to masculinity, and, importantly, it has been seen as the subordinate term in this dichotomy. Traits associated with masculinity tend to be culturally valorized, while those associated with femininity are subordinated. Fashion allows us to see this quite clearly: the qualities associated with it, including superficiality and artifice, are maligned while their masculinized opposites—depth and authenticity—constitute foundational social values in the West. Thus, the ways in which fashion gets mapped onto women reflect dichotomous regimes of gender, and can also reinforce and help to produce these regimes. After all, fashion is a lived cultural construct; its proximity to women's bodies is crucial, this volume shows, in reproducing the naturalization of dichotomous gender—as well as in challenging such reproductions.

Already it should be clear from this definition that there is a range of femininities, only a few of which are captured in this volume. Norms and thus practices of femininity vary, of course, according to social variables such as class, sexuality, ethnicity, and nation. We hope to signal this diversity through our titular invocation of the multiple *cultures* of femininity, which produce multiple feminine affects and practices. As these essays show, the flexibility of the concept has produced, in modernity, a rich and textured range of ways to instantiate femininity, even as the construct coalesces around several overarching normative concepts.

Fashion, Femininity, and Feminist Theory

Many more recent scholars of fashion and modernity—including Evans, Lehmann, and Wilson—have complicated long-standing associations between fashion and femininity by pointing out fashion's ubiquity and widespread influence on modernity in its multiple guises. In addition, scholars including Christopher Breward have examined men's engagement with changing styles of dress in the nineteenth and twentieth centuries.[9] Such work has helped to recover fashion from the realm of the frivolous and the ephemeral and has greatly advanced our understanding of dress's important place in accounts of modern culture and society. Yet having recognized fashion's broader reach, our volume demonstrates that it is necessary and productive to return to the connection between fashion and femininity as a point of articulation that must be further interrogated rather than assumed or rejected. By recognizing the ways in which fashion was gendered in the period we study, this collection seeks to better understand the relationship between all three concepts—fashion, femininity, and modernity—in order to place gender at the forefront of accounts of both fashion and modernity. Femininity shifts and consolidates in the late nineteenth and early twentieth centuries, in part through fashion. The gendered phenomenon of fashion reflects and reinscribes women's conceptual and material associations with spectacle, matter, consumption, mutability, irrationality, and conformity. It also provides a conditional site for negotiating and challenging such frameworks of gender.

Certainly feminist work in modernist studies has brought increased attention to the centrality of women in the cultural consciousness of the modern. Yet explicit attention to fashion could make that point even clearer—and it could do so by bringing out the affective dimensions of the condition of modern womanhood. Scholarship on images of women illuminates the representational dimensions of this phenomenon: it mines the periodical press and advertising archives, for instance, for visual and textual imagery to show how women bore the meaning of the modern. But it does not get us very far in reconstructing what it might have been like for women to embody modernity, what it felt like to become modern and to experience the self as modern. As a number of the essays in this volume show, fashion can help to deliver us the missing piece: the piece that entails the modern woman's own recognition and fashioning of self-identity. What did buying, touching, making, and wearing clothing suggest to these women about the stakes of being modern?

To address this question, the collection examines women's experiences as consumers, designers, and critics of fashion, incorporating accounts of fashion from photographs, diaries, letters, periodicals, and literature. Celia Marshik's chapter, for example, investigates women's engagement with fashionability through the archives of a secondhand clothing dealer in Britain in the early twentieth century, while Christina Bates explores the intimate experience and political significance of wearing different styles of nurses' uniforms in late nineteenth-century Canada. Such work suggests a new direction for further inquiries into the relationship between women and modernity, as fashion allows us to analyze public spectacles of femininity and intimate mediations of dress in the everyday and psychic lives of women. By integrating the individual and social dimensions of women's identities, fashion disrupts the tendency to reproduce static and ontologizing characterizations of the modern woman. In foregrounding the way collective and individual selves produce and reproduce each other in the course of a modern life, fashion can help us to see the continual, processual emergence of femininity as a defining feature of the modern, one that is inextricable from the public cultures of modernity. Such work goes some of the way toward undoing the public and private divide that has been challenged in feminist history and theory, but which still exists in some iterations of modernist studies, art history, and literary studies; scholarship in these fields often attends to the arts and the public culture of modernism without delving very deeply into the way these draw on and inform the everyday lives of ostensibly private citizens. To this end, the chapter by Jasmine Rault shows how architect Eileen Gray drew upon the ambiguous boundary between secret and spectacle in 1920s "lesbian" fashion to imagine simultaneously private and public spaces, which made room for alternative constructions of gender and sexuality.

In addition to taking up feminist theory's challenge to the division between public and private, this volume approaches the study of fashion as a bridge between conceptual divisions that continue to concern feminist scholars. In particular, the collection intervenes in theoretical impasses in feminist theory by showing that fashion functioned as a join between the discursive and material dimensions of modern life. In attending simultaneously to the conditions that produced femininity and the lived experiences of fashion, many of the essays contribute to an emergent feminist materialism that interrogates the divide between materialism and poststructuralism.[10] Elizabeth Sheehan's chapter on the studio photography of James VanDerZee in Harlem in the 1920s and 1930s, and a chapter by Kimberly Wahl on the wearing of the tea gown in artistic circles in late nineteenth-century London, for example, shed new light on the connections between the material and discursive construction of feminine identities. Through such work, fashion comes into view as an integrative medium, bringing together public and private, intimate and spectacular, individual and collective, as well as material and conceptual.

Cultures of Femininity

Fashion's integrative and multiple nature can be expressed through the idea of "cultures of femininity," which guides this volume. This approach treats affiliations among women—or the barriers to those affiliations—as a central object of analysis. In doing so, it can convey to us the tensions—or, sometimes, the convergences—between individual enactments of femininity and collective fantasies of womanhood; see, for example, Ellen Bayuk Rosenman and Kara Tennant's chapters on the discourses and practices of fashionable Victorian femininity. It also draws upon a rich history of feminist interrogations of the primacy of the individual masculinist subject to suggest that the more compelling narratives of what it meant to be modern can be found in dialogic spaces. They are more compelling because they are noisier stories, full of multivalent conversations and conflicts. They are also more compelling because, as this volume suggests, they capture the aspects of life as a modern subject that are overlooked by analyses that posit the central struggle of the modern as an interior one.

Other work has challenged this focus on the individual in modernity. Yet, although there has been great interest recently in transnational affiliations and in collectivities invoked by and responding to mass culture and mass politics, less attention has been given to collective gender formation, affiliation, and disaffiliation. This volume's focus on cultures of femininity brings forward such concerns in part by attending to the seemingly more pedestrian sphere of the everyday—from drawing rooms to dress shops to family photographs and personal letters—rather than the monumental. In doing so we resist what Rita Felski has shown is the gendered binary between enriching public time and deadening daily time. As Felski observes, this dismissal of the everyday reinforces the idea that women—identified with the mundane—are seen to dwell in "habitual, home-centered spaces [that] are outside, and in some sense antithetical to, the experience of an authentic modernity."[11] Fashion offers a different vision of the everyday. As social theorists of fashion make clear, it is a large part of what makes everyday life dynamic. Because changing clothing involved micrological shifts in how modern subjects forged their individual identities through and against other subjects and collectivities, it was part of what made modern daily life vital, changeable.

It is also important to remember that fashion was crucial in naturalizing feminine spectacle in everyday life; that is, women in this period came to embody spectacle, as they were conceived as the primary consumers of fashion and as they mediated dress and fashion in their daily lives.[12] Thus, fashion systems, while they were integrated into everyday lives, also orchestrated public spectacles, as Justine De Young demonstrates in her discussion of the paintings in the Paris Salon of 1868. This connection destabilizes the tired binary between daily time and monumental time that has proved so hostile to conceiving of women's modernity. Fashion can thus show us how identity is forged in the spaces of everyday life, and how this is a continually ongoing and contested process. It can redescribe everyday life in ways that center it—and, by extension, women—at the heart of the modern.

Fashion also helps us see everyday life as a site for identity formation through both self-perceptions and negotiations of the self in relation to others, as individuals position themselves within and through the cultures of femininity this volume highlights. Fashion provides the ground for an analysis of collectivities as dynamic and dissonant entities that are composed of individuals—that central category in modernity—whose selfhood is formed through interactions with other people, communities, objects, and ideas. To this end, chapters by Elizabeth Sheehan and Lori Harrison-Kahan examine how fashion invokes gendered and racialized discourses of communal and individual identity.

In a 2003 paper on the relationships between cultural studies and modernist studies, Rita Felski points to the importance of that old standby in cultural studies, the concept of articulation, which she describes as a "theory of social correspondences, non-correspondences, and contradictions."[13] This idea of articulation applies to this volume's account of fashion in two senses: first, the collected essays show how fashion became a site of connections and conflict between various concepts—such as modernity and femininity, professionalism and domesticity—in the modern imaginary. Christina Bates, for instance, uses the example of nursing uniforms to show that fashion was a point of articulation for emerging concepts of professionalism and discourses of femininity. The volume also brings to light connections or articulations among individuals as they make up larger communities of thought and action in the era of industrial modernity.

In order to explore fashion as a site of articulation, the collection brings together a variety of disciplinary and methodological approaches. Academic institutions are currently clamoring for more interdisciplinary work. The chapters show the need for and benefits of such integrated approaches by demonstrating that the phenomenon of fashion is best understood through diverse disciplinary lenses. As our volume shows, fashion was a pivotal aspect of modern periodical culture, material culture, visual culture, and even literature, and hence its place in modern culture can be comprehended only by using such a multi- and interdisciplinary approach. In turn, by bringing together work by specialists in art history, literature, history, American studies, cultural studies, and curation, the collection demonstrates that an analysis of fashion can enrich how an array of disciplines theorize modernity and femininity. In particular, a number of the chapters, including Lori Harrison-Kahan's, Kara Tennant's, and Ellen Bayuk Rosenman's, address the relatively neglected topic of dress and fashion within studies of modern literature. Certainly the volume's unifying focus on the connections and barriers among women is a question that is more often treated in social scientific literature. In describing these articulations from the perspective of literature, art history, and historical analysis, the essays collected here highlight the permeability of the barrier between social scientific and humanistic approaches to the question of the modern.[14]

Of course, our focus on gendered collectivities is hardly unprecedented; there is certainly a literature on the formation of modernist intellectual and artistic circles in various cities in the early twentieth century. There is also a specific literature on groups of women modernists; Shari Benstock's work on communities of artistic women on Paris's Left Bank is a good example.[15] What is missing, for the most part, is a detailed analysis of the constitution of cultures of femininity that does not rest wholly on the retrieval of the history of groups of modern women, nor altogether on the discursive mediations of femininity in the popular press, advertising, or the cinema. What we need—or need much more of, because Laura Doan's book on the origins of modern English lesbian culture is a rare example[16]—is a literature on women and modernity that can account for the simultaneously discursive and experiential material dimensions of life as a gendered, modern subject. Foregrounding the cultures of femininity through fashion can do precisely such productive and important work, which refuses to fragment these dimensions and thus challenges the ongoing positioning of women as desiccated modern puppets.

Fashion can do this for us because the fashion system—to use Roland Barthes's term[17]—is a simultaneously discursive and material construct, one that engages the symbolic and lived dimensions of human experience and makes clear to us the inextricability of these dimensions. It can help us do the work of identifying and analyzing these cultures of femininity as textured, conflicted, collective, and always embodied sites, without trivializing or dismissing the psychic, affective, and imaginative dimensions of modern life as a gendered subject. It can do this for us because it is a kind of hybrid, which complicates the easy dichotomization of individual and collective fantasy, private and public time, and conceptual and experiential mediations of the modern.

The multifariousness and ubiquity of fashion helps us not only to overcome gendered binaries that persist in the study of modernity, but also to trace the diverse contours of modernity and femininity across time, space, and cultural difference. Simultaneously global and local, collective and individual, fashion brings to light connections among diverse cultures of femininity from mid-Victorian London to early twentieth-century Harlem in this volume. At the same time, fashion is a visual and material sign of the persistent differences that serve to interrupt universalizing accounts of modernity or femininity. Dress makes visible the distinctions in the ways that cultures of femininity developed within the diverse material, temporal, and cultural conditions of modernity. One contribution this collection seeks to make is to show the ways in which fashion generates intersecting norms and practices of femininity in diverse national contexts, including Britain, the United States, France, and Canada.

Fashion is a particularly effective way to trace both shared and unique aspects of various cultures of femininity in modernity, in part because there is an ongoing debate in costume history as to whether modernity has brought about a democratization or continued stratification of fashion. As scholars have noted, the spread of consumer culture made fashion more available and more visible to a wider swath of the population, and some costume historians have described fashion as becoming increasingly "democratized" beginning in the mid-to-late nineteenth century.[18] As several of the essays in this volume illustrate, some art, fiction, and periodicals of the period depict fashion as blurring or obscuring class, ethnic, and gender identity. In this sense, dress appears to provide the means through which individuals and communities could negotiate and manipulate the shifting terrain of modern selfhood. Such a reading also suggests that fashion could provide symbolic and physical material that would enable imagined cultures of femininity to stretch across such differences. Yet, as many of the chapters demonstrate, there is also ample evidence of the ways that fashion consolidated social divisions. After all, clothing remained a sign of difference and its availability remained highly uneven and variable.[19] New fashions in many ways altered and created, rather than erased, the visual vocabulary of class, ethnic, and racial difference. This volume takes up both of these strands of dress history to show that fashion uncovers similarities and disjunctions in how femininity was conceived and experienced in the era of industrial modernity.

Organization of the Volume

The collected essays are grouped along several thematic axes that pivot on the question of how fashion shaped cultures of femininity in modernity. The sections span several different national contexts and historical periods as they underline the transhistorical and transnational applicability of a "cultures of femininity" approach, without homogenizing the very specific circumstances it treats. The first section of the book highlights the importance of fashion in both the establishment and the breakdown of collectivities of women in the late nineteenth and early twentieth century. Jasmine Rault, in "Fashioning Sapphic Architecture: Eileen Gray and Radclyffe Hall," makes a uniquely interdisciplinary contribution with her discussion of the relationship between the ambiguous aesthetics used in architect and interior designer Eileen Gray's work, and the complex sartorial codes used by communities of wealthy "lesbian" women in the 1920s. In "A Domesticated Exoticism: Fashioning Gender in Nineteenth-Century British Tea Gowns," Kimberly Wahl argues that the tea gown was a kind of hybrid garment, embodying the conflicting but mutually dependent meanings of modernism and antimodernism, and establishing groups of middle- and upper-middle-class artistic British women as ambiguously modern subjects through the gowns' Orientalist underpinnings. Together, Rault and Wahl's analyses call us to attend to the ways that fashion, though on one level an intensely individualist medium, was also central to the formation of communities of women in the modern period. Wahl's essay in particular also attends to the class and racial exclusions upon which such fashions—and, in turn, such cultures of femininity—depended.

As fashion materializes the mutually constitutive relationship between individual and community, it also makes visible the tensions that characterize collectivities of women; after all, the impulse to distinguish the self sartorially was very often at odds with the cultivation of broader collectives. In the other essay in this section, dress and fashion are shown not only to catalyze in the formation of cultures of modern femininity, but also to create barriers to affiliations among women. Celia Marshik's "Smart Clothes at Low Prices: Alliances and Negotiations in the British Interwar Secondhand Clothing Trade" examines the correspondence of a second-hand clothing dealer, Robina Wallis, illustrating the fraught negotiations of class and status that occurred when women ostensibly came together over fashion in the 1920s through the 1940s. Even as this volume seeks to foreground the relationships among women in the modern period, fash-ion acts as a corrective to the tendency to idealize those connections and ignore the very real differences that existed among women. The resultant account of stresses within these cultures of femininity shows these cul-tures to be complex and conflicted.

The volume's second section delves deeper into the issue of class, showing how fashion as a realm of feminine expertise and practice cut across and consolidated social boundaries. The chapters here build on the existing literature about women and consumption, which has explored how women's status as consumers facilitated their access to the public sphere beginning in the mid-nineteenth century, sometimes leading to panic about the transgression of social orders. Each chapter adds depth and material specificity to this scholarship by showing how these cultural tensions played out in embodied interactions with dressed women, as fashionable clothing was linked to anxieties about the agency of middle-class women in a rapidly developing urban consumer culture. Ellen Bayuk Rosenman's "Fear of Fashion; or, How the Coquette Got Her Bad Name" stresses the ways that fashion was seen to establish for women in Victorian England a realm of knowledge and expertise that lent them a certain autonomy from men. Also treating Victorian England, Kara Ten-nant, in "The Discerning Eye: Viewing the Mid-Victorian 'Modern' Woman," analyzes the periodical press and popular literature to argue that the wearing of fashionable dress made visual identification of wom-en's status difficult, leading to fears about the threat posed by the "mod-ern" to established class and gender orders. In "'Housewife or Harlot': Art, Fashion, and Morality in the Paris Salon of 1868," Justine De Young traces a similar debate in the same period in France, offering a detailed reading of the moral dimensions of the anxious critical response to Charles-François Marchal's paintings of fashionably dressed women at the 1868 Paris Salon. Focusing on the way that fashionable dress, specifi-cally, was related to questions of visuality and popular knowledge—what could be known about women, and what remained hidden, as a result of their visible sartorial practices?—the essays in this section add a fresh epistemological dimension to the literature in this area.

Moving from the visual to the material dimension of women's lives, the volume's third and final section brings together examples from disparate times and places, showing how central dress was to gendered, raced, and classed embodiment in the modern period. In "'Their Uniforms all Esthetic and Antiseptic': Fashioning Modern Nursing Identity, 1870–1900," Christina Bates contributes a nuanced reading of nursing uniforms in several late nineteenth-century Canadian contexts; as a specialist in material culture, she begins with the objects themselves to build a history of this developing feminized labor force and of modern Canadian women's experience more broadly. In "The Face of Fashion: Race and Fantasy in James VanDerZee's Photography and Jessie Fauset's Fiction," Elizabeth Sheehan describes fashion as a site of tension and negotiation between material and imaginary constructions of race and gender in early twentieth-century Harlem. Lori Harrison-Kahan's "'More Than a Garment': Edna Ferber and the Fashioning of Transnational Identity" offers a reading of Edna Ferber's fiction to illustrate how the matter of dress interweaves different discourses of identity, including masculinity and femininity, Jewishness and Americanness, leisure class and working class. What emerges is a sense of the garments in remaking ideas and practices of womanhood in the context of women's professionalization and movements for gender and racial justice.

Together the essays collected in this volume show that fashion was much more than a reflection of ideas about femininity in late nineteenth- and early twentieth-century Western culture. Rather, fashion helped to create cultures of modern femininity in both the popular imagination and the everyday practices of women's lives. By recovering fashion as a dynamic and far-reaching force in modern culture and politics, the volume discovers a nuanced, dialogic, and conflicted terrain of femininity during the late nineteenth and early twentieth centuries. Demonstrating fashion's inextricability from modern life, the volume also argues for placing gender, everyday life, and materiality at the forefront of our accounts of modernity. Grounded in the ubiquitous, ever-changing matter of fashion, *Cultures of Femininity in Modern Fashion* places women at the heart of modern culture, as its agents and exemplars.

Notes

1. Kathy Peiss, "Girls Lean Back Everywhere," in *The Modern Girl Around the World: Consumption, Modernity, and Globalization*, ed. The Modern Girl Around the World Research Group (Durham, NC: Duke University Press, 2008), 351.

2. Andreas Huyssen, *After the Great Divide: Modernism, Mass Culture, Postmodernism* (New York: Columbia University Press, 1986); Rita Felski, *The Gender of Modernity* (Cambridge, MA: Harvard University Press, 1995); Marshall Berman, *All That Is Solid Melts into Air: The Experience of Modernity* (New York: Simon and Schuster, 1982).

3. See Michel Foucault, *The Order of Things: An Archaeology of the Human Sciences* [1966] (New York: Random House, 1970), and Harvie Ferguson, *Modernity and Subjectivity: Body, Soul, Spirit* (Charlottesville: University of Virginia Press, 2000).

4. Dilip Parameshwar Gaonkar, "On Alternative Modernities," *Public Culture* 11, no. 1 (1999): 16.

5. Georg Simmel, "The Philosophy of Fashion," [1905] in *Simmel on Culture*, ed. David Frisby and Mike Featherstone (London: Sage, 1997). Walter Benjamin, "Paris, Capital of the Nineteenth Century," [1939] in *The Arcades Project*, trans. Howard Eiland and Kevin McLaughlin (Cambridge, MA: Belknap Press, 2000).

6. Charles Baudelaire, "The Painter of Modern Life," [1863] in *The Painter of Modern Life and Other Essays*, trans. Jonathan Mayne (London: Phaidon Press, 1964), 12.

7. Elizabeth Wilson, *Adorned in Dreams: Fashion and Modernity*, rev. ed. (New Brunswick, NJ: Rutgers University Press, 2003); Elizabeth Wilson, "Fashion in Modernity," in *Fashion and Modernity*, ed. Christopher Breward and Caroline Evans (Oxford: Berg, 2005); Ulrich Lehmann, *Tigersprung: Fashion in Modernity* (Cambridge, MA: MIT Press, 2000); Caroline Evans, *Fashion at the Edge: Spectacle, Modernity, and Deathliness* (Cambridge, MA: MIT Press, 2003).

8. Judith Butler, *Gender Trouble* (London and New York: Routledge, 1990); and *Bodies That Matter* (London and New York: Routledge, 1993).

9. Christopher Breward, *The Hidden Consumer: Masculinities, Fashion, and City Life, 1860–1914* (Manchester, UK: Manchester University Press, 1999).

10. For a representative work in this vein, see the collection *Material Feminisms*, ed. Stacey Alaimo and Susan Hekman (Bloomington: Indiana University Press, 2008).

11. Rita Felski, "The Invention of Everyday Life," in *Doing Time: Feminist Theory and Postmodern Culture* (New York: New York University Press, 2000), 81.

12. On the question of the naturalization and feminization of spectacle in the late nineteenth and early twentieth centuries, see Abigail Solomon-Godeau, "The Other Side of Venus: The Visual Economy of Feminine Display," in *The Sex of Things: Gender and Consumption in Historical Perspective*, ed. Victoria de Grazia (Berkeley: University of California Press, 1996), and Liz Conor, *The Spectacular Modern Woman: Feminine Visibility in the 1920s* (Bloomington: Indiana University Press, 2004).

13. Rita Felski, "Modernist Studies and Cultural Studies: Reflections on Method," *Modernism/Modernity* 10, no. 3 (2003): 511.

14. For an illuminating discussion of the divide between the humanities and the social sciences in modernist studies, see Susan Stanford Friedman, "Definitional Exclusions: The Meaning of Modern/Modernity/Modernism," *Modernism/Modernity* 8, no. 3 (2001): 493–513.

15. Shari Benstock, *Women of the Left Bank* (Austin: University of Texas Press, 1987).

16. Laura Doan, *Fashioning Sapphism: The Origins of Modern English Lesbian Culture* (New York: Columbia University Press, 2001).

17. Roland Barthes, *The Fashion System* [1967], trans. Matthew Ward and Richard Howard (New York: Hill and Wang, 1983).

18. A representative example is Elizabeth Ewing, *History of Twentieth Century Fashion*, rev. ed. (London: Batsford, 2001). See also Martine Elzingre, *Femmes habillées. La mode de luxe: styles et images* (Paris: Austral, 1996).

19. Diana Crane and Philippe Perrot are among those who refute the democratization thesis. Diana Crane, *Fashion and its Social Agendas: Class, Gender, and Identity in Clothing* (Chicago: University of Chicago Press, 2000); Philippe Perrot, *Fashioning the Bourgeoisie: A History of Clothing in the Nineteenth Century*, trans. Richard Bienvenu (Princeton: Princeton University Press, 1994).

FASHION AND RELATIONSHIPS AMONG MODERN WOMEN

🌿 I

FASHIONING SAPPHIC ARCHITECTURE

Eileen Gray and Radclyffe Hall

When you are surrounded with shadows and dark corners you are at
home only as far as the hazy edges of the darkness your eyes cannot
penetrate. You are not master in your own house.
—Le Corbusier

External architecture seems to have absorbed avant-garde architects at
the expense of the interior, as if a house should be conceived for the
pleasure of the eye more than for the well-being of its inhabitants.
—Eileen Gray

The same roof mustn't shelter us both any more.
—Radclyffe Hall

What would it mean to read Eileen Gray's intricately designed, first
built house, E.1027 (1928), as an architectural elaboration of sapphic fashion? This involves exploring the possibility that Gray, who has
been read as an isolated figure, an exceptional woman among great masters,
was both influenced by and contributed to a culture of non-heterosexual
female modernity from which Gray scholars have been careful to distance
her.[1] It also offers to the literature on fashion and modern architecture
an increased attention to the historical and cultural specificity of sartorial
styles themselves. Mark Wigley has persuasively argued that modern architecture was "haunted by the spectre of fashion."[2] But to make sense of
Gray's work, we need to ask which fashions. Historians of sapphic modernity have shown that the popularity of mannish female fashions during the 1920s in France and England enabled some women—mostly white,
upper and upper-middle class women—to cultivate modes of female

masculinity that ambiguously communicated both new-woman chic and same-sex desire.[3] If historians of architecture and fashion miss the specific historical, cultural, and erotic significance of this ambiguous look, we risk missing the significance of the architectures it enabled. This essay thus shifts the conventional terms of engagement with Gray's work by reading it into a cultural history of sapphic modernity, demonstrates the importance of attending to the specificity of the fashions that influenced modern architecture, and hopes ultimately to open new lines of inquiry for feminist accounts of female sexual dissidence in early twentieth-century visual and architectural modernity. But first, we need to start with the story of E.1027.

In 1928, after nearly twenty years of working in interior design in Paris and about four years spent informally studying architecture, Gray completed her first house, E.1027, on an isolated oceanfront plot of land in the south of France. By 1938, Le Corbusier, perhaps the most influential figure in European modernist architecture, had painted a total of eight murals on the walls of E.1027—making a mark on Gray's work that would literally not be erased (figure 1.1).[4] Gray's biographer writes of the mural painting as an act of sexual violence: "It was a rape. A fellow architect, a man she admired, had without her consent defaced her design."[5] Le Corbusier's uncanny interest in her house led him, in 1952, to build himself a small hut on E.1027's property line, directly overlooking her space. He would eventually come to occupy the site, living out his last eight years there before drowning in the waters off its shore. Beatriz Colomina first told this story in 1993, where she suggests that Le Corbusier's peculiar "war" on Gray's architecture was related to both her gender and her non-heterosexuality.[6] My own research on Gray has been motivated by the question of what there was in her architecture and design that compelled Le Corbusier's obsessive, invasive, and sexualized violence? And to what extent has Le Corbusier's initial heteronormative violence marked and continued to structure critical perspectives on Gray's work?

This essay attempts to address these questions by offering an alternative perspective on E.1027, one that is guided by Gray's own efforts there to develop other ways of looking. While Colomina suggests that Le Corbusier's violence was related in some way to the fact that Gray was "openly gay,"[7] alternative or non-heterosexual female sexualities in the 1920s had not yet accrued into such a stable cultural or social identity. Gray's sexuality, despite her reputed intimate relationships with women and with her architectural tutor, Jean Badovici, would not have looked like anything we recognize as lesbian, bisexual, or heterosexual.[8] Women like Gray who lived outside the bounds of conventional heterosexuality

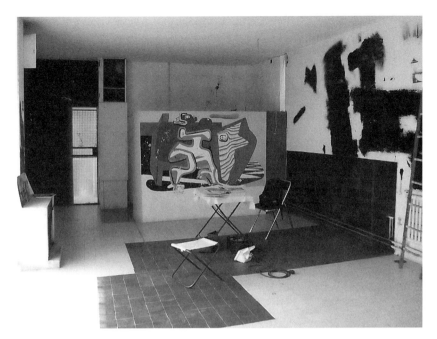

in the 1920s were not yet clearly or unambiguously recognizable or identifiable, which historians have suggested played a role in their representational strategies, or in their efforts to create alternative ways of looking—of both appearing and seeing.[9] Moreover, with the risks of social and cultural persecution and legal prosecution, sexually dissident women's other ways of looking were fundamentally and necessarily ambiguous, straddling the volatile line between revealing and concealing what was seen as a culturally deviant, medically degenerate, and increasingly criminal desire. These are some of the concerns for women in the 1920s that would have structured what Annamarie Jagose has described as "the ambivalent relationship between the lesbian and the field of vision,"[10] which importantly informed women's fashions and carefully ambiguous self-fashionings, and which I hope to show influenced the critical visual strategies that Gray used at E.1027.

E.1027 was completed the same year that Radclyffe Hall published what tends to be considered the first lesbian novel, *The Well of Loneliness* (1928), where the quest for appropriate domestic space is at the center of the problem of non-heterosexual identity.[11] Stephen Gordon, Hall's semi-autobiographical heroine in *The Well*, is exiled from her aristocratic family home, Morton House, and spends the rest of the novel in search of a shelter for her sexual identity and relationships. Everything she does from the time of exile is in the service of creating domestic space appropriate to homosexual desire and subjectivity—and she doggedly pursues a writing career as a "shelter" (346) for herself and her lover. Through Stephen, Hall proposes a model of non-heterosexual female subjectivity whose only chance for survival is to create appropriate domestic space—and whose aesthetic work is conceived as primarily architectural. Those elements that Gray argues are missing from modern architecture turn out to be the very same as those for which Stephen is searching. Comparing E.1027 to *The Well of Loneliness* suggests the extent to which architecture and interior design were understood to be implicated in constitutions of non-heterosexuality in the 1920s, and, moreover, that Gray was invested in building homes for sexual exiles like Stephen.

I want to suggest that sapphic fashions played an important role in the critical alternative Gray offered with E.1027 to the dynamics and erotics of vision, of total exposure, exteriority, and the pleasure of visual mastery, which Le Corbusier had defined and influentially promoted throughout the 1920s. I argue that Gray designed E.1027 for the kind of sexual and gender dissidents who Hall asserted, in *The Well*, were denied appropriate living space in the 1920s, and that Gray's critically different visual dynamics are related to the erotics of visual ambiguity that non-heterosexual women cultivated through their masculinized self-fashionings in the 1920s—a visibility based, like Gray's designs, on ambivalence, suggestion, partial views, and glimpses, as much on concealing as revealing. I contend that Hall is significant to understandings of E.1027; first, because her novel dramatizes non-heterosexual women's need for living spaces like those that Gray designed, and, second, because just as Le Corbusier is central to understanding the visual dynamics and the primacy of vision in modern architecture, Hall is central to understanding the sartorial and visual dynamics cultivated by female sexual dissidents in the 1920s, and the eventual reduction of these ambiguous dynamics to a fixed and circumscribed image of lesbian identity.

In the context of this volume, my chapter might be understood as an exploration less of "cultures of femininity" than cultures of female masculinities, both sartorial and architectural. The modern cultures of female masculinities that I explore here challenge the assumption of any one modern culture of femininity and complement this volume's interest in denaturalizing the relationships between femininity and female bodies, as well as femininity and fashion. Modern fashions in female masculinity in the 1920s enabled a kind of ambiguity that both suggested and protected gender and sexual dissidence—which was also the sort of enabling ambiguity achieved in female appropriations of conventionally masculinized private space. That is, feminist theorists and architectural historians have shown that, despite normative assumptions and assertions of the gendered division between public and private spheres, the only privacy that women have conventionally secured in domestic space has been men's (specifically, white, heterosexual, upper-middle- and upper-class men's privacy).[12] The cultivation of masculinity in fashions and architecture for female subjects created spaces of possibility for dissident embodiments and inhabitations of gender and sexual ambiguity.

Recent studies in sapphic modernity have shown that understanding such gender and sexual dissidence is central to understanding early twentieth-century European modernity. As Joanne Winning argues, what constituted the *modern* of any modern identity at the time was the tension of a non-identitarian sexual dissident becoming "a mixture of possibility and closure, dissolution and formation, excitement and terror. . . . [T]o be sapphist is *indelibly* to be modern."[13] That is, the unhinged sapphic sexual dynamism and tension constituted the modern's promise of becoming and futurity. This chapter can be understood as an exploration of the sapphic fashions that informed sapphic architecture at a moment in history before the excitement and possibility of ambiguous gender and sexual dissidence was closed and formed into a reductive modern architectural image and lesbian sexual identity.

Modernity, since the mid-nineteenth century, has been characterized by shifting modes of vision and a new emphasis on visuality generally.[14] And vision, perhaps more than anything else, was at the heart of Le Corbusier's modernist project. In 1923, he articulates this project most succinctly when he declares that modernist architecture is fundamentally about "RE-WARDING THE DESIRE OF OUR EYES."[15] Le Corbusier promoted a modernist architectural program that was based on stripping and exposure—removing a building's ornamental, decorative clothing and revealing its pure, truthful, naked body. Central to this visual program was white paint: "Put on it anything dishonest or in bad taste—it hits you in the eye. It is rather like an X-ray of beauty . . . It is the eye of truth."[16] The whiteness that would become the definitive look of modern architecture was first defined and promoted by Le Corbusier in *L'art décoratif d'aujourd'hui* (1925), where he invites the reader to join in his fantasy of Ripolin (whitewash):

Imagine the results of the Law of Ripolin. Every citizen is required to replace his hangings, his damasks, his wallpapers, his stencils, with a plain coat of white ripolin. *His home is made clean.* There are no more dirty, dark corners. *Everything is shown as it is.* When you are surrounded with shadows and dark corners you are at home only as far as the hazy edges of the darkness your eyes cannot penetrate. You are not master in your own house.[17]

Le Corbusier led the modernist architectural investment in whitewash as a form of uncovering, of stripping off the dishonest, ornamental garb to reveal the essential truth, showing "everything as it is." Mark Wigley explains that it was in 1927, at the *Weissenhofsiedlung* exhibition in Austria, when architects and designers from across Europe reached an "unprecedented . . . level of agreement about white,"[18] that modern architecture first came to be: "The exhibition . . . facilitated the reduction of the diverse tendencies and contradictions of the avant-garde into a recognizable 'look.'"[19] Early twentieth-century architecture and design became a modern movement and international style in the moment that it agreed on one unifying and reductive look.

The reductive look that came to be definitive of modern architecture, however, needs to be understood as both an appearance and a way of seeing. Colomina explains that "[s]eeing, for Le Corbusier, is the primordial activity of the house. The house is a device to see the world, a mechanism for viewing."[20] As Wigley puts it, his houses are "[n]ot machines for looking at but machines for looking."[21] Moreover, when it comes to understanding the look, and the looking, of Le Corbusier's architectural modernity, "fashion is the key."[22] It turns out that both the appearance of his architecture and the viewing of it promised were importantly modeled on men's and women's fashions in clothing. And if we turn to Le Corbusier's writing on clothing, we can get a sense of the strongly hetero-gendered dynamics built into this look. When not mired in color, decoration, and ornament "suited to simple races, peasants, and savages,"[23] new women's fashions, for example, demonstrate the modernist architectural principle of exposure. He praises women's dress reforms as modernist innovations in uncovering:

woman cut her hair and her skirts and her sleeves. She goes out bareheaded, bare armed, with her legs free. . . . And she is beautiful; she seduces us with the charm of her graces. . . . The courage, the liveliness, the spirit of invention with which woman has revolutionized her dress are a miracle of modern times. Thank you![24]

Modern architecture stripped of ornament promises the same obvious visual pleasures as female bodies stripped of clothing. Women's modern revolutions offered new visual technologies of seductive exposure. Le Corbusier reports the seductions of women's dresses as lessons in modernity:

The women are beautiful to behold, beautifully coiffured even in the harsh light and all decked out in exquisite dresses. To us they are not like strangers whose costumes alone would create a barrier ... all these things urged us to notice and admire them.[25]

Modern women's dress is no longer a barrier. It is an invitation to men's notice and admiration. Men's dress, by contrast, erases the male body: "It had *neutralized* us. . . . The dominant sign is no longer ostrich feathers in the hat, it is in the gaze. That's enough."[26] Here, Le Corbusier borrows directly from Adolf Loos, who had explained that "modern man needs his clothes as a mask."[27] The clothes to which they refer are specifically those which comprise the "English suit we wear" and this man's suit figures prominently in visions of architectural modernity. As Wigley points out, Le Corbusier situates this "well-cut suit," "plain jacket," and "smooth white shirt" at the center of his visual and architectural project, "acting as the link between the modernization of industrial culture that has already occurred and the modernization of architectural culture that is about to occur."[28] Modern architecture offered the same revolutionary visual dynamics found in modern fashion, whereby men enjoy the invisible authority and pleasure of looking at exposed female bodies, and women enjoy the modern sensation of always being looked at by men.

Gray's architecture, like her fashion, disrupted this distinctly hetero-gendered visual dynamic. Like the women Le Corbusier admired, Gray did cut her hair short, and she may have cut her skirts, but she was remembered "wearing a trouser suit and a neat bow tie."[29] Indeed, like many women in the 1920s, Gray's fashion choices tended more toward the masculinized layers of Le Corbusier's well-cut suit than the feminized stripping that seduced him. The only photographs of Gray from the late 1920s that have survived were taken by Berenice Abbott in 1926 (figure 1.2).[30] Gray's cropped hair, smooth, high-collared white shirt, and plain tailored jacket signal both Gray's claim to and disturbance of Le Corbusier's vision of modernity. That is, her look would have communicated both the modern female fashion reform that Le Corbusier enjoyed and the queered female masculinity that was given no place in modernist architecture. These photographs, taken by the woman with a reputation for photographing "high culture's Left Bank lesbian set of the 1920s,"[31] show that Gray's strategies for masculinized self-fashioning correspond to those cultivated by many of her non-heterosexual female contemporaries—including several of Abbott's portrait subjects (such as Edna St. Vincent Millay, Janet Flanner, Jane Heap, and Sylvia Beach), Romaine Brooks and her painted portrait subjects (such as Una Troubridge, Gluck, and Renata

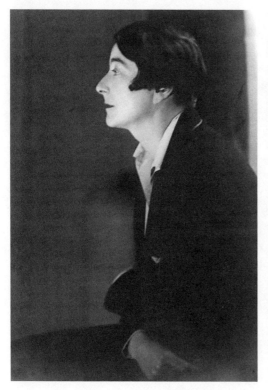

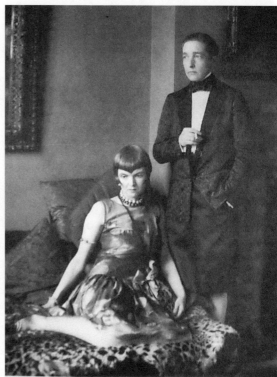

Figure 1.2 Eileen Gray, photograph by Berenice Abbott, 1926. *Courtesy of the National Museum of Ireland.* (Plate 2.)

Figure 1.3 Radclyffe Hall and Una Troubridge at home, 1926. *Fox Photos.*

Borgatti), and of course Radclyffe Hall. While Hall fashioned a much more formal, conservative, upper-class British masculinity than Gray (figure 1.3)—as we can see in this carefully staged photograph of her and her partner Lady Una Troubridge at their home in 1927, with her short and shining Eton crop, her gentleman's velvet evening jacket buttoned closed, her pressed white shirt collar tied—they both cultivated styles of female masculinity that have been read as telltale signs of lesbianism. However, recent historians of modernity and sexuality have argued convincingly that this look was not so straightforwardly revealing.

Gray's masculinized fashions would have straddled the line between outré new woman fashion and upper-class mannish lesbian. Indeed, a study on modern fashions of female femininity would be incomplete without considering the massive popularity of fashions in female masculinity at the time. Paris in the 1920s saw an explosion of simplified, gender-blurring *mode à la garçonne*, popularized famously by designers like Coco Chanel and Paul Poiret and hairstylists like René Rambaud; and at the same time, London witnessed the rising popularity of the "boyette" or the "masculine note" in female fashions.[32] Journalists, politicians, doctors, architects, and all forms of social and cultural commentators in both London and Paris were preoccupied by women's changing fashion in the 1920s. As Mary Louise Roberts explains, "[f]ashion bore the symbolic weight of a whole set of social anxieties concerning ... gender relations: the blurring or reversal of gender boundaries and the crisis of domesticity."[33] Reactions to women's tendency to "disguise themselves as men" ranged from laudatory to humorous to insulting:

Postwar critics spoke of a certain absence or lack of definition, which characterized both the new female body and "womanhood" itself. They interpreted the fashions that the modern woman wore as reproducing her inability to be defined within the boundaries of traditional concepts of womanhood.[34]

Roberts points out, not incidentally, that this anxiety was informed by scientific discourse on sexual inversion "inspired by the translation of Havelock Ellis into French. 'The species feels itself endangered by a growing inversion,' the literary critic Pierre Lièvre argued in 1927, 'no more hips, no more breasts, no more hair.'"[35] The discourse of dangerous inversion would have resonated by the 1920s with sexological descriptions of female homosexuality. Krafft-Ebing writes, for example, that "[female inversion] may nearly always be suspected in females wearing their hair short, or who dress in the fashion of men, or pursue the sports and pastimes of their male acquaintances;" such women exhibit "masculine features ... manly gait ... [and] small breasts."[36] Havelock Ellis focused less on physical characteristics than taste: the female invert can be detected in "traits of masculine simplicity ... [and] frequently a pronounced taste for smoking cigarettes ... also a decided taste and toleration for cigars."[37] Female homosexuality, they argued, could be either indicated or created by taking on the mannerisms, professions, hobbies, fashions, or desires of men. Masculinized fashions, critics feared, were masculinizing women, which according to the scientifically informed logic of the time resulted in lesbianism.

However, not all critics, and not all women, would have read these new masculinized fashions as indications of female sexual inversion. In her study of early twentieth-century British lesbian culture, Doan looks at

the pervasive phenomenon of masculine fashion for women, with its concomitant openness and fluidity, to explore the ways in which some women, primarily of the upper middle and upper classes, exploit the ambiguity that tolerated, even encouraged, the crossing over of fixed labels and assigned categories such as female boy, woman of fashion in the masculine mode, lesbian boy, mannish lesbian, and female cross-dresser.[38]

The visual codes around masculinized femininity were not yet fixed in the 1920s, and while some would recognize its implications of female sexual inversion (the mannish lesbian), this was not its only or necessarily primary meaning. Doan focuses on Hall's notoriously masculine fashions to show that while she tends to be read by today's viewers as typifying lesbian style, "it is important to remember that [she] appeared quite differently to the press and public in the 1920s."[39] Hall was a major figure in the upper classes of artistic London nightlife in the 1920s, and rather than being taken as the visual epitome of a sexually deviant subculture, she was invariably read as the vanguard of chic modern style. For example, after receiving the prestigious Femina Prize for her 1926 novel *Adam's Breed*, photos of Hall were featured in newspapers throughout England praising her for being "in the front rank of . . . modern fashions in dress."[40] As the widely circulated 1927 photograph of Hall and Troubridge suggests (figure 1.3), while certain viewers were undoubtedly familiar with the inverted sexual implications of her mannish look, uppermiddle and upper-class artistic women like Hall were able to enjoy the ambiguity of such masculinized female fashions to simultaneously reveal and conceal their non-heterosexuality. Doan describes the visual dynamics of such fashions:

Before public exposure, for the better part of a decade, masculine-style clothing for women held diverse spectatorial effects, with few signifiers giving the game away, and readings (whether of clothing, visual images, or stories about women living with other women in "close companionship") varied accordingly among those who knew, those who knew nothing, and those who wished they didn't know.[41]

That is, in 1926 and 1927, Gray's masculinized fashion, like Hall's, was as much a way of concealing or "neutralizing" same-sex desire as it was a means of showing it or rendering it visible. Gray's look, unlike Le Corbusier's, was necessarily ambiguous. And this ambiguity troubled heteromasculinist assumptions of the access that Le Corbusier saw promised by fashions in female femininity.

Gray cultivated, like Hall and many of their female contemporaries, a sartorial disruption to the distinctly heteronormative visual pleasure promised by Le Corbusier's architecture—the pleasure of concealed, invisible men watching exposed, always visible women. If we turn now to E.1027, we can see that Gray's architecture followed the logic of fashion no less, but quite differently, than Le Corbusier's. Gray appears to have taken part in those fashion reforms that Le Corbusier praised, just as she took part in those architectural reforms, but rather than celebrating their power to show and reveal, she seems to have capitalized on their potential to do the opposite, to obstruct and evoke.

Gray seems to have designed E.1027 as a critique of the visual agenda built into Le Corbusier's houses in the 1920s. In her only published writing, included in the special 1929 issue of *L'Architecture Vivante* dedicated to E.1027, Gray observes that "[e]xternal architecture seems to have absorbed avant-garde architects at the expense of the interior, as if a house should be conceived for the pleasure of the eye more than for the well-being of its inhabitants" (240). In marked contrast to Le Corbusier's desire for the visual pleasure of total exposure, modern architecture's definitive desire, Gray writes that

the interior should respond to human needs and the exigencies of individual life, and it should ensure calm and intimacy ... by interpreting the desires, passions, and tastes of the individual. . . . [A house] is not just the expression of abstract relationships; it must also encapsulate the most tangible relations, the most intimate needs of subjective life. (240, 239)

Gray designed for intimate needs, desires, passions, and tastes that were not entirely visible, the existence of which depended on the possibility of invisibility. As Constant explains, "[i]ntertwining the visible with what is out of sight, she manipulated vision to different ends. . . . Gray sought to transcend the reductive nature of the total view."[42] Even in a "house of restricted dimensions" (241), she explains, inhabitants "must have the *impression* of being alone, and if desired, entirely alone" (241).[43] Despite having adopted Le Corbusier's "free plan"—which he advocated in a 1927 issue of *L'Architecture Vivante* for its capacity to open domestic space before the spectator as a vista, a total view—Gray designed several strategies to obstruct the absolute visibility it promised and ensure the possibility of privacy, even in a relatively open space.[44]

The house consists of two bedrooms and a large central living room adjoined by a small alcove, all which are intended to serve as separate living/sleeping areas.[45] Gray's photographs emphasize the independence of every area, even when they provide glimpses through to adjoining rooms. The photograph of the main living room, for example, shows a darkly shadowed area sunken into the wall at the back (*top left corner*, figure 1.4). While we can see that this area, the sleeping alcove, is not structurally separate from the main room, Gray created the impression of separation by closing the shutters on both windows that would have lit the area, above the alcove's divan and on its door to the side deck. She photographs the alcove itself separately, with a close-up image of the divan's wall-mounted headrest with electrical outlets, reading lights, and bedside table, the open book and comfortably compressed, creased cushion emphasizing the privacy and intimacy that she hoped to secure in even this relatively exposed niche.

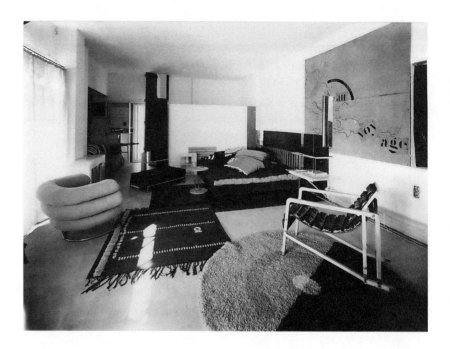

Gray was particularly attentive to thresholds between spaces, to doors and entrances. She writes, "One avoids making a door when one fears that it may open at any moment, evoking the possibility of an inopportune visit.... This has led us to position the walls so that the doors remain out of sight" (241). The floor plan shows that the privacy of each space is protected through sunken doors that open into the room—so that when one enters, their view of the room is blocked by both the open door and the wall into which it is sunk, delaying a visitor's visual access until the point that they are physically enmeshed in the space they see. Throughout E.1027, Gray designed screening devices, sunken doors, hidden by partial walls, extended by storage partitions, which worked to obstruct the reductive pleasure of total visibility and protect the privacy of each area of the house.

Gray's insistence on securing a conventionally masculinized privilege of privacy for each inhabitant, and in each area, needs to be understood as a radical challenge to the gendered order of things in 1929. This was, of course, the year that Virginia Woolf made the daring and controversial assertion that the possibility of doing creative work was predicated on this exclusively male privilege to a room of one's own, or "that a lock on the door means the power to think for oneself."[46] While only one room (off the main bedroom) was entitled "boudoir/studio," each separate living area was designed for this dual purpose, "merging" as Caroline Constant notes, "the historically gendered spaces of boudoir and study into a single entity."[47] The living room, alcove, and two bedrooms are each equipped with a bed or divan, a bedside reading light and storage space for books, adjustable, at times built-in pivoting, bedside tables for reading and writing, and a separate exit to the deck or garden.[48] Gray's merging of gendered domestic space was indeed unprecedented in the work of her avant-garde contemporaries,[49] and her interest in ensuring for potentially female inhabitants the masculinized privacy of a study brings us to considering some of the important ways that E.1027 was designed to accommodate such characters as Hall's Stephen Gordon.

In *The Well of Loneliness*, the space of the study is inextricably linked to the realization of female masculinity and non-heterosexuality. When Stephen's "unnatural" (203) sexual desire for another woman is exposed to her mother's "terrible eyes, pitiless and deeply accusing" (202), she retreats first to her father's study. In the moment when Stephen most needs to "claim an understanding" of her unnatural and unwanted self, she is naturally drawn "by some natal instinct" to the house's most potent architectural symbol of masculinity, to the locked secrets of her father's study.[50] But instead of the familiarity and comfort that it once offered, her father's study renders her alienation more acute as she recognizes that the protection the study secures is for the masculinity that she has no natural right to. Inside the locked bookcase in her father's private study, Stephen finds the answer to "the riddle of her unwanted being" (206) in the work of Richard von Krafft-Ebing, the first sexologist to name and study sexual inversion, the term for homosexuality at the time. The study turns out to be the room where the secret of her masculinity and unnatural desire is locked up as well as where it is revealed. Stephen goes on in the novel to build two more studies, sheltering these books and the more or less open secret of her masculinity. Victoria Rosner argues that in *The Well*, and in other novels at the time, "[m]asculinity hinges on privacy to such a marked extent that when women in these texts acquire their own private spaces, they become masculine ... the possession of culturally masculine attributes [like a private study] is often understood as the possession of hidden biological ones."[51] These dynamics of hiding and "coming out," of concealing and revealing a sexual secret, are symbolized in the *The Well* by the study or private domestic space, and turn out to be the same dynamics and architectural spaces that E.1027 addresses.

Stephen is a writer who conceives of her literary work in architectural terms. When Stephen's lover, Mary, worries over Stephen's long and taxing hours of writing, Stephen reasons, "I'm trying to build you a shelter" (346), and goes back to her work. As Rosner argues, Stephen longs to build a shelter that was unlike the architecture she knew—unlike that architecture which operated "as a regimented theatre of control in which women are typically confined to interior spaces, heterosexual desire alone is granted shelter, and exteriority is privileged over interiority."[52] Like Gray, Stephen hopes to build a home that will shelter her private tastes, intimacies, and desires—a house that grants protection from the "terrible, pitiless and deeply accusing eyes" that had banished her. The only other domestic space where Stephen feels comfortable is at the house of Valérie Seymour, a character that Hall based on Natalie Barney, who hosted famous weekly salons from her house on Rue Jacob, just around the corner from Gray's apartment in Paris.[53] "The first thing that struck Stephen about Valérie's flat was its large and rather splendid disorder. There was something blissfully unkempt about it . . . Nothing was quite where it ought to have been, and much was where it ought not to have been, while over the whole lay a faint layer of dust" (246). This "splendid disorder" was the heart of homosexual high culture and community in pre- and interwar Paris, both in Hall's novel and her life. To the stream of exiles that flowed into Paris, "the shipwrecked, the drowning . . . poor spluttering victims" (356), Valérie/Barney offered "the freedom" and "the protection . . . of her salon" (356). As Rosner explains, "Valérie's rooms offer a fully developed alternative to the domesticity of Morton . . . a gorgeous mess that permits gender categories to blend and blur, a place where such blurring seems the rule rather than the taboo exception."[54] The dust and disorder provides an alternative not only to Morton, but also to the fantasy of total hygiene propagated by modern architecture at the time.

As Colomina has explained, modernist architecture conceived of itself as "a kind of medical equipment," securing both hygienic domestic spaces and hygienic bodies.[55] Modernist architecture, to recall Le Corbusier, was medical equipment geared to purge the dusty disorder, the blurred boundaries and hazy edges that make exiles like Stephen feel brave and protected. Colomina argues that the modern house is "first and foremost a machine for health, a form of therapy,"[56] but the first sign of health for Le Corbusier was "*to love purity!*"[57] This conception of architectural-therapeutic purity provided literally no room for figures like Stephen, who were understood according to the medical logic at the time as fundamentally mixed: as Krafft-Ebing put it, "[t]he masculine soul, heaving in the female bosom,"[58] or, as Hall puts it, "mid-way between the sexes" (81). Modernist architecture's health and hygiene campaign was aimed specifically at "blissfully unkempt" houses like Valérie's and may have registered as a threat to those who personified the disorder it was meant to treat. "Yes!" Gray writes, "We will be killed by hygiene."[59] While perhaps lacking in dust, we can see among the tousled throw cushions and blankets, overlapping wool carpets, and toppled pile of magazines in Gray's photograph of E.1027's living room the sort of blissfully unkempt, or splendid disarray that Hall appreciated (see figure 1.4). Gray is less interested in clarifying those hazy or blurred edges that threaten the master of the house than in accommodating, cultivating, and enjoying them.

In Gray's private papers we can find rough notes that suggest that she was highly sensitive to the dynamics of desire and vision and that she designed to challenge the reductive tendencies of visual pleasure. She writes, for example, "la chicane sans donner une impression de résistance arrive le désir de pénétrer. donne la transition. garde le mystère. les objets à voir tiens en haleine le plaisir."[60] Gray admits of the desire of the eye, but is less interested in its satisfaction than its obstruction or deflection. Her photograph of the entryway partition suggests the effect that this obstructive visual strategy would have had (figure 1.5)—prolonging one's physical access to the room and breaking up the visual field into partial glimpses, both revealing and concealing, separating while still suggesting the porosity and connectivity of the spaces, provoking, as she explains, a desire for the sight to be seen. That is, she is interested in objects that remain just tantalizingly out of view, that keep their mystery, which withhold the satisfaction of total visibility or complete exposure and prolong the pleasure of desire itself. On the same page of notes, she writes that "the poverty of architecture today results from the atrophy of sensuality."[61] Judging from the lines just preceding this intriguing criticism, it seems that sensuality for Gray was constituted by the play between exposure and concealment, between seeing and the desire to see.

The pleasure of Gray's design and architecture takes place on the cusp between the visible and the invisible. In another page of notes on "interior architecture" (Architecture Intérieure), she writes of

La tristesse des 2 voyageurs entrant dans la salle à manger de l'hôtel aux 200 couverts éternellement mis.

La femme éternellement parée.

Le monde extérieur—les gens—l'Art—ne valent que par leur pouvoir de suggérer.[62]

This is the only explicit reference to woman that I have ever seen in Gray's writing. And the term "parée" can be taken several ways. It can be "dressed up," "prepared," "ready to go," or simply "ready,"[63] and its meaning

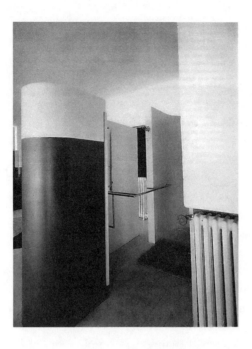

Figure 1.5 E.1027 entryway partition, with partial views through to living room, ca. 1928. Photograph by Eileen Gray. *Courtesy of the National Museum of Ireland.*

depends on the phrase it follows and continues. Gray imagines the sadness of travelers greeted by tables eternally set, by a room that loses its power to suggest the pleasures of a meal, of respite, rest, satiation, or satisfaction by its eagerness to fully expose itself. As though to reveal her point, to clarify, Gray uses the example of this ambiguously dressed-up, ready, or ready-to-go woman. We can assume that this woman, like the dining room, has lost her power to suggest some kind of pleasure through overexposure. All the same, Gray's point remains unclear. But by looking through her personal and published writings, as well as her designs of E.1027, this lack of clarity appears to *be* the point. She builds emphatically against the clarity that modern architecture most values, and toward the power of suggestion that the woman could embody if not for her total exposure. The eternally ready woman serves to illustrate the importance of ambiguity, of keeping something back, of not "showing everything as it is" according to Le Corbusier's fantasies.

These notes make it into Gray's published writing. In "De l'éclectisme au doute" she insists that "[e]very work of art is symbolic. It conveys, it suggests the essential more than representing it" (238). However, when Gray speaks of "the essential" she means something quite different than Le Corbusier's abstractly determined standard. Gray's essential is less universal than it is particular and contingent. It is an expression of "individual pleasures" that are determined by "the conditions of existence, of human tastes and aspirations, passions and needs" (238). The essential elements that structure Gray's architecture would be ruined by the total exposure that Le Corbusier advocates. Gray builds to suggest these individualized pleasures, passions, and needs, not to show them. Gray's assertion that the pleasure of private intimacies should trump the pleasure of seeing would have resonated beyond the confines of architectural debate and into the wider domain of social debates about fashion, gender, and sexuality, which, as Wigley and Colomina argue, sustain these architectural rhetorics of vision. The modernist architectural movement promoted by Le Corbusier was based on fashion, and indeed, if we are in search of a source for Gray's fundamentally ambiguous look, built into the furnishings and architecture of E.1027 and signaled in Gray's notes by the woman whose power of suggestion rests on her remaining on the cusp between the visible and the invisible, we can find it in new women's fashion in the 1920s.

In the 1920s, Hall and Gray's preferred look, like Gray's architecture and design, eschewed the absolute visibility and clear intelligibility that Le Corbusier praised. When Le Corbusier celebrated the visual pleasures of new women's fashion in the 1920s, he may have been referring to the same look that women like Hall and Gray favored. These innovations were embraced, however, by women like Gray and Hall less for their ability to reveal than their power to suggest. Tirza True Latimer explains that,

[in] the process of formulating image-making strategies capable of both communicating and dissimulating same-sex desires, lesbians of the early twentieth century confronted a number of interrelated dilemmas bearing on what Annamarie Jagose has described as "the ambivalent relationship between the lesbian and the field of vision."[64]

With the threat of social, cultural, and, in England, legal persecution, lesbians in the early twentieth century were compelled to cultivate what Latimer terms a "visible invisibility"—they could, of course, be seen, but only by those who knew how (and where) to look.[65] Marjorie Garber explains that "vestimentary codes" are a complex "system of signification":

[They] speak in a number of registers: class, gender, sexuality, erotic style. Part of the problem—and part of the pleasure and danger of decoding—is in determining which set of referents is in play in each scenario. For decoding itself is an erotics—in fact, one of the most powerful we know.[66]

This elaborate process of decoding, of learning how to look, constituted the pleasure (and danger) of sapphic visibility at the time—obviously and necessarily a very different erotics of vision than that which was promoted by Le Corbusier and modern architecture in the 1920s. However, the erotic dynamic of visible invisibility is significantly very similar to Gray's architectural investment in obstructing views to produce desire, or to her assertion that "the objects to be seen keep pleasure in suspense."[67]

Doan explains that through such sartorial codes lesbians in the 1920s entered into a uniquely ambivalent field of visibility, such that, "one woman's risk was another woman's opportunity, for *within* a discreet, perhaps miniscule, subculture, lesbians passed as stylishly recognizable lesbians as well as women of fashion."[68] However, the flexibility of these codes, Doan argues, was abruptly fixed at the time of Hall's obscenity trials in 1928. Within weeks of Hall's publication of the first "long and very serious novel entirely upon the subject of sexual inversion,"[69] the *Sunday Express* published a sensational attack on the book, which spearheaded the legal campaign against it. Most scholars have read these obscenity trials as demonstration that "the very suggestion of lesbian sexuality was enough to unleash remarkable animosity,"[70] or as examples of "hostility towards lesbianism."[71] However, Doan shows that in the years, and even days, preceding the article and the legal battle, lesbianism was not yet a stable point of reference against which the press, the public, or the courts could reasonably rail. Instead, the proliferation of photographs of Hall in the daily papers and the legal campaign associating her with "a particular hideous aspect of life as it exists among us today,"[72] from August to December of 1928, effectively created a lesbian identity modeled on Hall's previously stylish modern image. Post-1928, "[t]he very fashions that facilitated 'passing' in an earlier era would thus thrust some lesbians out into the open."[73] The photograph of Hall and Troubridge at home, for example, was carefully cropped for newspaper publications during the obscenity trials—cut just above Hall's knees, converting her stylish skirt to transgressive trousers, and removing Troubridge altogether, transforming the image of Hall from chic, fashionably skirt-suited new woman to the picture of deviant and criminal mannish lesbian (figure 1.6). After the trials, Hall's and thus Gray's masculinized look had lost much of its ambiguity and the dangers of being unequivocally "out in the open" were vividly pronounced in the press.

Considering Gray's only published statements about her work in light of the trials that had just six months before found Hall's novel obscene—a novel which is in part a plea for the creation of private domestic space

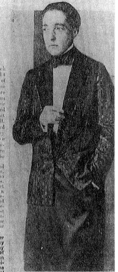

that would shelter atypical, non-heterosexual intimacies and desires—allows us to recognize some of the wider implications of Gray's criticisms of modernist architecture and "the pleasure of the eye." The story of E.1027, like all of Gray's work, has until very recently followed strictly heteronormative narrative lines: as a turning point in her maturation from decadent, figurative, and excessively personal decorative arts, which were conceived in early experimental relationships with women, to "pure" modernist, generalized, abstract architecture conceived in serious personal and professional relationships with modern masters.[74] Caroline Constant was the first to explore the critical edge to Gray's sensually engaging design and architecture[75] and Beatriz Colomina suggests that this critical sensuality was related to Gray's sexuality, which was in turn related to the sustained and sexualized disciplinary action by Le Corbusier, in the form of vandalism, occupation, and the eventual effacement of Gray's name and work. Despite Colomina's claims that "Gray was openly gay,"[76] it is not clear just how open Gray's gayness was. Save for this one unequivocal assertion, Gray's non-heterosexuality seems to have operated as a sort of open secret, as an erotics of visible invisibility in her work, her life, and in the literature that has struggled to make sense of her unaccountably critical sensuality. Indeed, Le Corbusier's visual philosophy of exposure would suggest that he hoped to reveal something that Gray had kept deliberately concealed. And his tripartite theory of muralling—to purify, to penetrate or enter, and to "violently destroy"[77]—suggests a desire to clarify the blurred and indefinite visibility that Gray cultivated, to forcibly insert himself into and so destroy an erotic dynamic that excluded or threatened him.

Colomina's version of the story of E.1027 suggests that the effacement of Gray's name and work from the history of modern architecture results from the systemic continuation of this first act of homophobic violence. We might think of Le Corbusier's effacement as a more successful censorship of homoerotic aesthetics than the one attempted by the London courts. The 1928 obscenity trials intruded on the privacy that Hall's ambiguous visibility had afforded her and reduced the erotically suggestive power of her image to an unambiguously identifiable and unacceptable "look," but ultimately boosted the international sales of her novel and secured her a place in the history books. In contrast, Le Corbusier's invasion of the privacy that Gray hoped to achieve with her erotically ambiguous visibility succeeded in concealing her work from view entirely for nearly forty years, so that by the time it was rediscovered, the sexually suggestive critical edge of her work was reduced to what the literature on her continues to consider a nearly unintelligible sensual engagement. Allowing Hall into the story of E.1027 lets us consider the relationship between Gray's critical emphases on suggestion, interiority, intimacy, individualized pleasures and privacy, the eroticized ambiguity of sapphic fashions and visual culture, and the heteronormative theoretical framework that has been sustained by editing these relationships out of histories of architectural modernity.

Notes

Le Corbusier, *The Decorative Art of Today* [1925] (Cambridge, MA: MIT Press, 1987): 188; emphasis in original.

Eileen Gray, "De l'éclecticisme au doute" ["From Eclecticism to Doubt"], in "Maison en bord de mer," *L'Architecture Vivante* (Winter 1929), translated in Caroline Constant, *Eileen Gray* (London: Phaidon Press Limited, 2000), 240. Gray published two articles: one entitled simply "Description" and the other, in the form of a dialogue between herself and Jean Badovici, entitled "De l'éclecticisme au doute," in "Maison en bord de mer," *L'Architecture Vivante* (Winter 1929), 17–35. Unless otherwise noted, all further references to Gray's published writings will come from the translation provided in Constant's *Eileen Gray*, 238–44.

Radclyffe Hall, *The Well of Loneliness* (London: Virago Press, Ltd., 1982), 205.

1. Efforts to align Gray with the "great masters" of modernist architecture, to insist upon her isolation and her distance from or rejection of other women, characterizes the majority of the literature on Gray, from the 1970s up to 2000, with the republication of Peter Adam's biography, and the publication of Caro-

line Constant's *Eileen Gray*. See Stewart Johnson, "Pioneer Lady," *Architectural Review*, 152 (August 1972); Joseph Rykwert, "Eileen Gray: Pioneer of Design," *Architectural Review* 152, no. 910 (December 1972); Joseph Rykwert, "Eileen Gray: Two Houses and an Interior, 1926–1933," *Perspecta*, 13/14 (1972); Reyner Banham, "Nostalgia for Style," *New Society* (February 1973); Peter Adam, *Eileen Gray: Architect, Designer, a Biography* (New York: Abrams, 2000). The tendency to read Gray as an isolated and/or pioneering woman has been repeated even in most feminist scholarship, with the exciting exception of Bridget Elliott's "Housing the Work: Women Artists, Modernism and the *Maison d'artiste*: Eileen Gray, Romaine Brooks, and Gluck," *Women Artists and the Decorative Arts, 1880–1935: The Gender of Ornament*, ed. Bridget Elliott and Janice Helland (Aldershot, England; Burlington, VT: Ashgate, 2002).

2. Mark Wigley, *White Walls, Designer Dresses: The Fashioning of Modern Architecture* (Cambridge, MA: MIT Press, 1995), 52.

3. See especially, Laura Doan, *Fashioning Sapphism: The Origins of a Modern English Lesbian Culture* (New York: Columbia University Press, 2001).

4. Until very recently, Gray's name, work, and especially her non-heterosexuality were absent from histories of modern architecture and design, and E.1027 has been deteriorating through years of neglect and vandalism. Photos of Le Corbusier's murals at E.1027 are published in *L'Architecture d'aujourd'hui* (April, 1948), with no mention of Gray. In an article entitled, "Le Corbusier, Muraliste," published in *Interiors* (June 1948), the caption to the murals at Roquebrune-Cap Martin not only leaves out Gray's name, but locates them "in a house designed by Le Corbusier and P. Jeanneret." In several publications between 1944 and 1981, E.1027 and its furnishings are attributed to Le Corbusier and/or Badovici (see Adam 2000, 334–35). By 2001, E.1027 had been declared a *monument historique* in France, but until 2007, E.1027 was still crumbling, restoration efforts stalled over the question of what to do with Le Corbusier's murals. As of 2008, work is finally underway to restore the house to its original 1928 condition, with the exception of the murals, which will remain.

5. Peter Adam, *Eileen Gray*, 311.

6. Beatriz Colomina, "War on Architecture," *Assemblage* 20 (1993), 28–29. This short article was republished at least three more times: Beatriz Colomina, "Battle Lines: E.1027," *Center*, no. 9, (1995): 22–31; Beatriz Colomina, "Battle Lines: E.1027," in *The Architect: Reconstructing Her Practice,* ed. F. Hughes (Cambridge, MA: MIT Press, 1996), 2–25; Beatriz Colomina, "Battle Lines: E.1027," in *The Sex of Architecture*, ed. Diana Agrest, Patricia Conway, Leslie Kanes Weisman (New York: Abrams, 1996), 167–90. Colomina also included an excerpt of this article in *Privacy and Publicity: Modern Architecture as Mass Media* [1994] (Cambridge, MA: MIT Press, 1998), 84–88. Moreover, as Colomina told me in conversation on July 11, 2004, the article has apparently been translated into at least four different languages. I have been able to find two published translations: "Lignes de bataille: E.1027," *Revue d'esthétique*, 29 (1996); "Frentes de batalla: E.1027," *Zehar*, 44 (2000): 8–13.

7. Colomina, "War On Architecture," 28.

8. Instead of reading a contemporary sexual identity back onto Gray, I would like to suggest with Lynne Walker that "[i]t seems less important what [Gray's]

sexual activities were than to try to explain the role that sexuality played in her creative life." Walker, "Architecture and Reputation: Eileen Gray, Gender, and Modernism," in *Women's Places: Architecture and Design 1860–1960*, ed. Brenda Martin and Penny Sparke (London and New York: Routledge, 2003), 104.

9. Joe Lucchesi, "'The Dandy in Me': Romaine Brooks's 1923 Portraits" in *Dandies: Fashion and Finesse in Art and Culture*, ed. Susan Fillin-Yeh (New York and London: New York University Press, 2001); Bridget Elliott, "Performing the Picture or Painting the Other: Romaine Brooks, Gluck, and the Question of Decadence in 1923" in *Women Artists and Modernism*, ed. Katy Deepwell (Manchester; New York: Manchester University Press, 1998); Bridget Elliott and Jo-Ann Wallace, *Women Artists and Writers: Modernist (im)positionings* (London; New York: Routledge, 1994); Laura Doan, *Fashioning Sapphism*; Tirza True Latimer, *Looking Like a Lesbian: The Sexual Politics of Portraiture in Paris Between the Wars* (PhD dissertation, Stanford University, 2002); Whitney Chadwick and Tirza True Latimer, "Introduction" and "Becoming Modern: Gender and Sexual Identity after World War I" in *The Modern Woman Revisited: Paris Between the Wars*, ed. Chadwick and Latimer (New Brunswick, NJ; London: Rutgers University Press, 2003); Tirza True Latimer, *Women Together/Women Apart: Portraits of Lesbian Paris* (New Brunswick; NJ: Rutgers University Press, 2005).

10. Annamarie Jagose, *Inconsequence: Lesbian Representation and the Logic of Sequence* (Ithaca, NY: Cornell University Press, 2002), 2.

11. While *The Well* has long been read as the first and prototypical literary representation of lesbianism—the cover of my edition dubs it "a classic story of lesbian love" (Virago Press Limited, 1994)—recent scholarship has shown that the term "lesbian" can only be retrospectively and at best uneasily applied to the main character, Stephen Gordon. Jay Prosser argues that Hall's description of Stephen's extreme gender dysphoria needs to be understood as the first narrative of transsexuality, before such a category existed (Prosser, *Second Skins: The Body Narratives of Transsexuality* [New York: Colombia University Press, 1998]), and Laura Doan argues that the lesbian identity which has so persistently been read back into Hall's story is an *effect* of the novel, its obscenity trials, and the photographic images of Hall that they became conflated with at the time (Doan, *Fashioning Sapphism: The Origins of a Modern English Lesbian Culture* [New York: Columbia University Press, 2001]). Indeed, the word "lesbian" is conspicuously absent from the novel, which relies instead on the sexologists' terminology of "inversion." Throughout the chapter, I have tried to use the term "invert" when discussing the novel, "non-heterosexual" or "homosexual" when discussing its implications for Gray's work and female subjectivities at the time, and "lesbian" as a post-1928 identity and theoretical perspective. All further references to the *Well of Loneliness* will come from Hall 1994.

12. For an excellent analysis of the architectural history of women as guardians of men's privacy, see Mark Wigley, "Housing Gender," in *Sexuality & Space*, ed. Beatriz Colomina and Jennifer Bloomer (New York: Princeton Architectural Press, 1992).

13. Joanne Winning, "The Sapphist in the City: Lesbian Modernist Paris and Sapphic Modernity," in *Sapphic Modernities: Sexuality, Women and National Culture*, ed. Laura Doan and Jane Garrity (New York: Palgrave Macmillan, 2006), 19.

14. For the history of modernity as a history of shifting visual perception, see Jonathan Crary, *Techniques of the Observer: On Vision and Modernity in the Nineteenth Century* (Cambridge, MA: MIT Press, 1990). For a feminist analysis of the gendered and sexualized history of vision and modernity, see Daryl Ogden, *The Language of the Eyes: Science, Sexuality, and Female Vision in English Literature and Culture, 1690–1927* (Albany: State University of New York Press, 2005). For some interesting essays on the role of fashion and display in nineteenth- and twentieth-century modernity, see Susan Fillin-Yeh, ed., *Dandies: Fashion and Finesse in Art and Culture* (New York and London: New York University Press, 2001).

15. Le Corbusier, *Towards a New Architecture* [1923], trans. F. Etchells (New York: Dover Publications, 1986), 16; emphases in original.

16. Le Corbusier, *The Decorative Art of Today* [1925], trans. James I. Dunnett (Cambridge, MA: MIT Press, 1987), 189.

17. Ibid., 188; emphasis in original.

18. Mark Wigley, *White Walls, Designer Dresses: The Fashioning of Modern Architecture* (Cambridge, MA: MIT Press, 1995), 302–303.

19. Ibid., 303.

20. Colomina, *Privacy and Publicity: Modern Architecture as Mass Media* (Cambridge, MA: MIT Press, 1998), 7.

21. Wigley, *White Walls*, 8.

22. Ibid., 52.

23. Le Corbusier, *Towards a New Architecture*, 143.

24. Le Corbusier, quoted in Colomina, *Privacy and Publicity*, 333–34.

25. Le Corbusier, quoted in Wigley, *White Walls*, 277.

26. Le Corbusier, quoted in Colomina, *Privacy and Publicity*, 334.

27. Adolf Loos, "Ornament and Crime," in *The Architecture of Adolf Loos: An Arts Council Exhibition*, trans. Wilfried Wang; ed. Yehuda Safran, Wilfried Wang, Mildred Budny (London: Arts Council of Great Britain, 1987), 103.

28. Wigley, *White Walls*, 17 (for Wigley's discussion of the role of the "generic man's suit" in Le Corbusier's architectural theory, see 16–18).

29. Peter Adam, reporting the recollections of Gray's carpenter at Tempe à Pailla, André-Joseph Roattino, *Eileen Gray*, 267–68.

30. Adam writes that Gray was photographed by Abbott again in 1927, but it remains unclear to me whether any of these photographs have survived (Adam, *Eileen Gray*, 185). In the Gray archives at the National Museum of Ireland, the photograph in figure 1.4 has "'26" noted below it. And while other very similar photographs in the archive have no date listed, Adam has dated them from 1926. It is possible that some of these photographs were taken in 1927, but this would mean that Gray had kept precisely the same hairstyle and length, and had donned the same outfit, down to the white handkerchief in her front jacket pocket. If this is the case, it seems Gray's carefully managed self-styling is all the more significant. However, it may be that the 1927 photographs are simply missing from Gray's available archives.

31. Laura Cottingham, referring to Berenice Abbott, in "Notes on Lesbian," *Art Journal*, 55, no. 4 (Winter 1996), 74.

32. On the political implications of boyish styles in France in the 1920s, see Mary Louise Roberts, "Samson and Delilah Revisited: The Politics of Fashion in

1920s France," in Chadwick and Latimer, *The Modern Woman Revisited*, 67–71. On the relationship between 1920s fashion and the creation of lesbian identities in England, see Doan, *Fashioning Sapphism*, particularly on the popularity of mannish female fashions, see 102–17.

33. Roberts Samson and Delilah, 67–68.

34. Ibid., 74.

35. Ibid., 74.

36. Richard von Krafft-Ebing, *Psychopathia Sexualis* [1886], reprinted in *Sexology Uncensored: The Documents of Sexual Science*, ed. Lucy Bland and Laura Doan (Chicago: The University of Chicago Press, 1989), 46.

37. Havelock Ellis, *Sexual Inversion* [1897], quoted in Doan, *Fashioning Sapphism*, 101.

38. Doan, *Fashioning Sapphism*, 99.

39. Ibid., 111.

40. From *Eve: The Ladies Pictorial*, July 13, 1927, quoted in Doan, *Fashioning Sapphism*, 110.

41. Laura Doan, *Fashioning Sapphism: The Origins of a Modern English Lesbian Culture* (New York: Columbia University Press, 2001), xiv.

42. Constant, *Eileen Gray*, 116–17.

43. The house is indeed relatively small: sixteen-hundred square feet on the upper level, twelve-hundred on the lower.

44. Le Corbusier, "Ou en est l'architecture?" in *L'Architecture Vivante* (Fall 1927).

45. The third room on the lower floor is the maid's room, "the *smallest habitable cell* . . . where one seeks only essential comfort" (244). This room is exceptionally smaller than any other in the house, and its essential comforts included only a bed and a washbasin, with one small window that is entirely blocked by an external *piloti*, or cement pillar. Gray writes that "this room could serve as an example of all rooms for children and servants" (244) and would indeed set the tone for her servant's room in the next two houses she built, reflecting a profoundly classist attitude to the maid, Louise Dany, with whom she would spend nearly fifty years of her life (1927–1976). Judging by Gray's letters, however, her relationship to Louise was more intimate and conflicted than her strictly separate architecture suggests.

46. Virginia Woolf, *A Room of One's Own* [1928] (London: HarperCollins, 1994), 115.

47. Constant, *Eileen Gray*, 107.

48. The divan in the alcove off the living room, for example, has, as Gray explained, "a flexible table with two pivots [which] allows for reading while lying down" (Gray, 242). This flexible table, built into the headrest with electrical sockets and reading lights on dimmer switches, was also used for Gray's bedroom in Paris.

49. For example, Le Corbusier's model house at the Pavillon de L'Esprit Nouveau (1925), Marcel Breuer's contribution to the Werkbund in Paris (1930), and Loos's Muller House in Prague (1930) all included separate rooms designated for the man and the woman of the house. As Bridget Elliott explains, unlike the avant-garde architecture upon which much of this first house was based, "Gray's solitary spaces were geared towards work and study [and I would add relaxing

and luxuriating] and not associated with either sex." Elliott, "Housing the Work: Women Artists, Modernism, and the *Maison d'artiste*: Eileen Gray, Romaine Brooks, and Gluck," in *Women Artists and the Decorative Arts, 1880–1935: The Gender of Ornament*, ed. Bridget Elliott and Janice Helland (England; Burlington, VT: Ashgate, 2002), 182.

50. "As though drawn there by some natal instinct, Stephen went straight to her father's study; and she sat in the old arm-chair that had survived him. . . . All the loneliness that had gone before was as nothing to this new loneliness of spirit. An immense desolation swept down upon her, an immense need to cry out and claim understanding for herself, an immense need to find an answer to the riddle of her unwanted being. All around her were grey and crumbling ruins, and under those ruins her love lay bleeding. . . . Getting up, she wandered about the room, touching its kind and familiar objects; stroking the desk, examining a pen . . . then she opened a little drawer in the desk and took out the key of her father's locked book-case" (205–206).

51. Rosner, *Housing Modernism*, 183–84.

52. Rosner, *Housing Modernism*, 29.

53. While Gray was an infrequent guest at Barney's events, in her 1929 *Aventures de L'Esprit*, Barney set a place for Gray at her table of esteemed friends. See frontisleaf to Natalie Barney, *Aventures de l'Esprit* (Paris: Éditions Émile-Paul Frères, 1929). And in 1919 and 1920, Barney sent Gray two books of her poetry, each with a personal inscription, which Gray kept throughout her life. Books of poetry by Barney are among her very few books at the Eileen Gray Archive, Collins Barracks, National Museum of Ireland.

54. Victoria Rosner, "Once More unto the Breach: *The Well of Loneliness* and the Spaces of Inversion," in *Palatable Poison: Critical Perspectives on* The Well of Loneliness, ed. Laura Doan and Jay Prosser (New York: Colombia University Press, 2001), 324.

55. Beatriz Colomina, "The Medical Body in Modern Architecture" in *Daidalos, Architektur, Kunst, Kultur* 64 (1997), 61.

56. Colomina, "The Medical Body," 64.

57. Le Corbusier, *The Decorative Art*, 188; italics in original.

58. Richard von Krafft-Ebing, *Psychopathia Sexualis* (1886), reprinted in *Sexology Uncensored: The Documents of Sexual Science*, ed. Lucy Bland and Laura Doan (Chicago: The University of Chicago Press, 1989), 47.

59. Gray, translated in Constant, *An Architecture for all Senses*, 70. In the original, Gray writes: "De l'hygiene à en mourir!" This 1996 translation seems more accurate than the 2000 version, which reads, "Hygiene to bore us to death!" (239).

60. "the deflector/divider without giving the impression of resistance brings the desire to penetrate. give the transition. keep the mystery. the objects to be seen keep pleasure in suspense." My translation, notes in the Gray archive, National Museum of Ireland.

61. "pauvreté de l'architecture d'aujourd'hui résultat de l'atrophie de la sensualité." My translation, notes in the Gray archive, National Museum of Ireland.

62. "The sadness of two travelers entering the dining room of a hotel to two hundred table settings eternally put out. / The woman eternally ready. / The ex-

terior world—people—Art—are valuable only by their power to suggest." Gray, "Architecture Intérieure," Gray archive, National Museum of Ireland.

63. *Collins Robert: Paperback French Dictionary* (Glasgow: HarperCollins Publishers, 1984).

64. Latimer, *Women Together/Women Apart* (New Brunswick, NJ: Rutgers University Press, 2005); 12, quoting Jagose, *Inconsequence*.

65. Latimer, *Women Together*, 12.

66. Marjorie Garber, *Vested Interests: Cross-Dressing and Cultural Anxiety* (New York: Routledge, 1992), 161.

67. Gray, notes in the Gray archive, National Museum of Ireland.

68. Doan, *Fashioning Sapphism*, 120.

69. Hall, quoted in Doan, *Fashioning Sapphism*, 1.

70. Joseph Bristow, 1997, quoted in Doan, *Fashioning Sapphism*, 4.

71. Deirdre Beddoe, 1989, quoted in Doan, *Fashioning Sapphism*, 4.

72. Douglas, 1928, quoted in Doan, *Fashioning Sapphism*, 18.

73. Ibid., 122.

74. Peter Adam writes that by the time Gray started working on E.1027, around 1926, she had entirely abandoned her earlier decorative art works—they were reminders of a life she had left far behind, "the sins of her youth" (375), and had begun to concentrate on "pure architecture" (147). Reiterating the narrative of Gray's life and career told by critics in the 1960s and 1970s, Adam's biography loosely aligns her aesthetically and sexually experimental youth with her decorative art and her serious, mature career with "pure architecture" and an intimate relationship to Badovici. Adam, *Eileen Gray*.

75. Constant, "E.1027: The Nonheroic Modernism of Eileen Gray," in *Journal of the Society of Architectural Historians* 25 (September 1994); Caroline Constant and Wilfried Wang, eds., *Eileen Gray: An Architecture for All Senses* (Wasmuth, MA: Harvard University Graduate School of Design, 1996).

76. Colomina, *Battle Lines*, 170.

77. Melony Ward explains that Le Corbusier understood his sketching and obsessive tracing and retracing of an image as a process of eliminating the excess, the unnecessary, and purifying an idea to its most essential form: "Drawing for Le Corbusier is a process of purification." Ward, "Cleaning House: Purity, Presence and the New Spirit in Le Corbusier," in *Practice Practise Praxis: Serial Repetition, Organizational Behaviour, and Strategic Action in Architecture*, ed. S. Sorli (Toronto: YYZ Books, 2000), 88. On entering, in *Creation is a Patient Search*, Le Corbusier writes, "By working with our hands, by drawing, we enter the house of a stranger" (Le Corbusier, *Creation*, 203). Finally, Le Corbusier explains in 1932, "I admit the mural not to enhance the wall, but on the contrary, as a means to violently destroy the wall, to remove from it all sense of stability, weight, etc." (Le Corbusier, from a letter to Vladimir Nekrassov, quoted in Colomina, *Battle Lines*, 174).

Kimberly Wahl

🌿 2

A DOMESTICATED EXOTICISM

Fashioning Gender in Nineteenth-Century British Tea Gowns

Victorian fashion has often been examined in terms of its regulation and control of the female body. The rules and rituals of fashionable dress have been perceived as limiting women's choices rather than enabling them. Work in the fields of fashion history and theory have complicated this picture, with scholars such as Elizabeth Wilson, Christopher Breward, Valerie Steele, and Joanne Entwistle all arguing that fashion, as an facet of material culture, allows women various degrees of self-expression, autonomy, and choice within a larger social sphere of physical and sartorial convention. Evidence for this may be found in a perusal of the fashion literature and visual culture of the late nineteenth century, which presents a rhetoric of freedom and self-expression addressed to a largely female readership. However, even analyses of late Victorian fashion that question accepted notions of containment and control have overlooked the destabilizing effects and subversive potential of Aestheticism, the degree to which the discourses of Orientalism shaped arguments about fashion and social decorum, and the resulting debates surrounding female sartorial creativity, autonomy, and choice. The Victorian tea gown, as the fashionable garment most impacted by British Aesthetic culture in the nineteenth century, was a unique form of dress wherein Aestheticism and Orientalism converged in important ways.

While few women wore Aesthetic dress publicly, many women indulged in exotic or artistic themes through the wearing of tea gowns, which were often cited in the fashion literature as a fashionable and comfortable mode of dress designed for use in the privacy of one's own home. The original function of the tea gown was to facilitate comfort and mobility, and it did not require corsets, crinolines, or bustles. Worn at tea time, between visiting or shopping trips and the formality of dinner, the tea gown was praised for allowing women forms of creativity and self-expression, often while hosting intimate get-togethers in a space of female leisure and comfort. Through artistic manifestations of the tea gown, experimentation and exploration of themes current in the art world were facilitated by the growing market of consumable goods from the East. The tea gown was especially valued for its ability to accommodate a wide range of styles; selected examples from the 1890 volume of *Woman's World* illustrate this diversity (figures 2.1 and 2.2). Heavily influenced by the historicism rampant throughout the Victorian period, various details of tea gowns point to a pronounced emphasis on past sartorial modes and exotic locales. In figure 2.1, the figure on the far left wears an Empire-waisted gown reminiscent of the early 1800s. Paired with this is a cloak with a high ruff collar, resembling styles popular in Europe at various times from the Renaissance through the seventeenth century. The figure on the far right wears a garment with an extra fabric panel extending to the floor from between the shoulder blades at the back. Referred to as a "Watteau panel" or "plait," this feature references eighteenth-century fashion and is closely tied to Aesthetic forms of dress in the 1870s and 1880s. In figure 2.2, the looseness of the gown, combined with its asymmetrical wrap closure, and overcoat/dress with short sleeves, are heavily influenced by the Orientalism of the period. Visual cues in the illustration underscore the gown's exoticism; the fan held by the wearer and the screen visible in the background both suggest an Aesthetic interior.

As one of the most visible and celebrated areas of late Victorian fashion, the tea gown was understood as a garment that empowered wearers through both creativity and comfort. Inflected by the artistic discourses of the Aesthetic movement, which favored dress reform principles, the tea gown gave women the opportunity to explore the margins of mainstream fashionable dress without an excess of social censure and public scrutiny, and was thus an outlet for self-expression and a potential means of resistance against mainstream cultural norms. The tea gown, when actually worn, was primarily viewed by an exclusive and rarefied audience—those invited into the privileged spaces of upper- and middle-class women's homes. This setting often guaranteed wearers a relatively sympathetic and appreciative audience. In addition, the flexibility and expressive qualities of the tea gown, as well as its prominence in the published fashion literature, signaled an active effort by some Victorian women to participate in the cycle of display, spectacle, and visual consumption that characterized the nineteenth-century urban experience of modernity. However, many proponents of design reform viewed Aesthetic dress as a

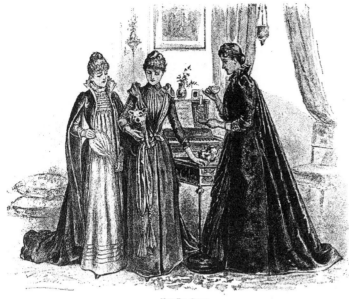

NEW TEA-GOWNS.

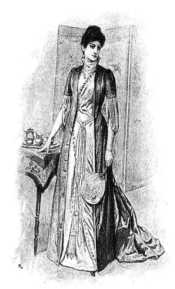

NEW TEA-GOWN.

timeless and stable prototype that might provide a more authentic alternative to the fickle and changeable nature of mainstream fashion. In this way, Aesthetic dress can be linked to the concurrent and more politicized dress reform movement of the period—a link that in and of itself establishes artistic dress as a form of social critique.

The growing popularity of the tea gown during this period points to its importance as a site of complex and often contradictory discourses surrounding notions of gender, space, and colonialism. By the 1880s, the link between Aesthetic dress and the "artistic" tea gown was firmly established, with themes of exoticism and antiquity prominent in the fashion literature as well as the visual arts. Paintings of the period feature artful arrangements of beautiful women lounging about in classical garb, and were carried out by artists such as Frederick Leighton, Alma Tadema, Albert Moore, and James McNeill Whistler. Sitters were often rendered exotic and sensual in appearance through the drapery and fabrics of either the distant past or the foreign East. Similar textiles, including sumptuous gauzes, fine silks, flowing muslins, and rare weaves, could be purchased at Liberty's in London, and were suggestive of imagination and fantasy. Encoded as foreign and strange, and also rare and exquisite, such fabrics cast the female wearer in the role of "other," and thus as exotic and desirable. Although the practice of Aesthetic dressing enabled women's sartorial choices, it simultaneously subjected women to a range of constraining social and artistic categories within Victorian artistic culture. For this

Figure 2.1 "New Tea Gowns." *Woman's World*, vol. 1 (London, 1890). *Courtesy of Queens University Stauffer Library.*

Figure 2.2 "New Tea-Gown." *Woman's World*, vol. 1 (London, 1890). *Courtesy of Queens University Stauffer Library.*

reason, the tea gown itself can also be viewed as a repository of social convention and meaning, suggesting the ideological containment of space, gender, and race.

The exoticism of the tea gown underscores its ambivalent relationship to modernity and illuminates the antimodern roots of Aesthetic art and culture.[1] Images of the distant past, the classical world, and the exotic "East" function as a foil for modern culture, and abound in the art and literature of Aestheticism; such references reveal the desire to engage with the cultural materials of "other" cultures as a possible antidote for the material and commercial concerns of modern living.[2] Further, the valorization of Eastern cultures through the gendered gaze of women involved with the Aesthetic movement points to a certain ambivalence within the visual culture of British imperialism. Reina Lewis has argued that women's artistic production in the late nineteenth century complicates traditional post-colonial critiques of Orientalism. Through an understanding of difference and a "gendered access to the positionalities of imperial discourse" women are in a unique position to view a colonial "other" "less pejoratively and less absolutely than was implied by Said's original formulation."[3] In the realm of fashion, other cultures served not only as a foil to which the fast-changing and innovative styles of modern culture might be compared, but provided inspiration, intrigue, and visual relief from the monotony and ubiquity of mainstream modes. In as much as the clothing associated with Eastern cultures might be viewed pejoratively by the Imperial project as traditional, antiquated, and even backward, such styles were also looked upon as a unique aesthetic and affective resource by artistic women in Victorian Britain.

This tension was felt in Aesthetic dress and other forms of artistic dressing popular in Britain during the late 1870s and early 1880s. The sartorial category of the tea gown was deeply influenced by conflicted, and, at times, contradictory themes, and this is evident when one closely examines contemporary forms of fashion communication—fashion plates, journalistic writing and reportage, and portraits of women in Aesthetic and/or artistic forms of dress heavily influenced by colonial narratives. This chapter assesses Orientalism's impact on the production of an artistic leisure culture for middle and upper-class women within the context of British Aestheticism. By examining how Orientalism shaped the representation and practice of wearing tea gowns, we can better understand the ideological function of fashion, not only as a form of social fantasy and play, but also in terms of how innovative or exploratory sartorial modes engaged with the codes of gender construction in Victorian cul-

ture. Ultimately, Aesthetic dress signaled an important space for the negotiation between the artistic discourses that bounded and/or enabled
female subjectivity and Imperial projections of an exotic "other" within
British Aestheticism.

Aesthetic Dress as an Embodied Social Practice

Before exploring the tea gown as a specific form of cultural address, an
understanding of Aesthetic dress as a mode of artistic production is required. Aesthetic forms of dress signified and shaped various constructions of femininity, where the perceived divide between high and low
cultural forms of Aesthetic art production and consumption were linked
with notions of female agency.[4] Juxtaposing these forms is a productive
way of examining the meaning and function of Aesthetic dress and the
degree to which it was empowering or limiting for women in the Aesthetic movement. The dominant explanatory model that contrasts high-
art Aesthetic production by male artists with derivative low-art appli-
cations in the realm of the decorative arts by craftspeople, and domestic
consumerism by women, is fraught with internal contradictions, even as
it is reified and supported in contemporary examples from the literature
on design reform. Regenia Gagnier and Kathy Alexis Psomiades have
interrogated this split by pointing out its ideological function in the service of gender construction and containment. Gagnier has argued that
the historical framing of Aestheticism denied the commodity nature of
art by foisting it outside the borders of artistic purity into a feminized
realm of popular culture.[5] For Psomiades, femininity itself became a useful trope within Aestheticism, signifying the double nature of art as apart
from the praxis of daily life while simultaneously commodified within
the marketplace; on one level Aestheticism is regarded as an autonomous
art form removed from daily life, and on another, it is necessarily commodified and disseminated in the proliferation of goods and services associated with an Aesthetic lifestyle.[6] An analysis of Aesthetic dress provides
a fruitful point of focus for several interrelated themes within Aesthetic
culture: female representation and subjectivity, the impact of artistic discourses on commercial goods within Aestheticism, and the consumable
images, objects, and other "spoils" of imperialism.

Many feminist analyses of Aestheticism have argued that women's role
in Aestheticism has not been sufficiently explored or researched. For both
Psomiades and Gagnier, the intentional distinction between productive
forms of Aestheticism and the consumption of Aesthetic culture obscures
the important contribution that women made to Aesthetic culture in the

closing years of the nineteenth century. I believe one way of addressing this problematic relationship is by mapping the absorption of alternative modes of dressing into mainstream fashion, and examining the inter-relation between popular and elite forms of Aesthetic dress. Rather than subscribing to the idea that high-culture forms and images of Aesthetic dressing were emulated by a passive populace, I would argue that Aesthetic dress was utilized, deployed, and ultimately recreated in the two spheres with varying results and intentions. Aesthetic dressing existed across a broad spectrum of artistic practices and enterprises. Just as a simple division between the production and consumption of Aestheticism is insufficient, so too a simple division between those forms donned by the artistic "insiders" of Aestheticism and more popular forms that emerged in consumer culture impedes a rigorous analysis of women's art production within Aestheticism and its significance for a wider audience of artistic culture. Aesthetic dressing provided an opportunity for women to consolidate and reconcile opposing formations of femininity within Aestheticism by allowing them to occupy a position as subject of Aesthetic sensibility and object of Aesthetic contemplation simultaneously. Further, in its active and performative function, Aesthetic dressing can, in some cases, be viewed as questioning, subverting, and even redressing the terms of female subjectivity within Aestheticism.

Through the fluid nature of commodity culture, the importation of Aesthetic dress into mainstream fashion allowed for a flowering of female creativity and agency in the marketplace of art-related goods. Erika Diane Rappaport and others have suggested that in the early years of the Victorian era the female shopper was a particularly disruptive figure, since a middle-class family's level of respectability and social position depended on the separation of the women in the household from the "filthy, fraudulent, and dangerous world of the urban marketplace." Increasingly, however, as public spaces catered more and more to respectable female consumers, shopping areas were progressive spaces for women and can therefore be seen as sites that, simultaneously and reproduced and disrupted established gender roles for women.[7] The nineteenth-century department store was characterized by fantasy and transformation; displayed items designed for private consumption can be seen as transitional objects—highly charged repositories of social meaning for the negotiation of gender and space. Consumer sites were thus liminal spaces where domestic and public identities lost their hard-edged boundaries.[8] The pleasure found in examining, choosing, and purchasing exquisite fabrics and other goods associated with the display of one's personal ideals of beauty would naturally have fed into the choices one made with regard to attire. Furthermore, the perceived ability of artistic goods to proclaim the advanced taste of those who bought them meant that commercial spaces took on an added importance for women who shopped for materials or ready-to-wear items associated with Aesthetic dress. Despite the anti-materialism expressed by purists within the Aesthetic movement, consumer culture can be credited with the dissemination of Aesthetic principles across a broader public spectrum; while women largely were denied entrance to many of the sanctioned realms of male creativity (painting, architecture, entrance to art academies), domestic forms of creativity typically gendered as "female," such as interior decorating and dressmaking, enabled many women, who otherwise would not have the opportunity, to express their artistic ideals.[9]

Women in Aesthetic circles were constantly surrounded by artistic representations of the female body, in private patrons' homes, or in gallery and exhibition spaces, and were thus implicated in a range of literary, mythic, and idyllic themes. As a consequence, the centrality of the female body as a signifying system within Aestheticism created an environment conducive to a heightened awareness of one's body as a physical presence in space. Through association or even identification, women within the Aesthetic movement would have been aware of themselves as objects of artistic contemplation and display. However, this understanding could not have completely obscured their experience of themselves as embodied subjects or their awareness of the agency they possessed with regard to the importance of the feminine in domestic Aesthetic settings. Elizabeth Wilson has argued that fashion can be empowering, particularly for the wearer, since it allows for an emphasis on beauty and the body in an ascetic and moralistic Judeo-Christian culture that has tended to belie or repress the sensuality of the body, particularly as expressed by women, for women.[10] Moreover, in Aesthetic dressing, the wearer might both construct herself as a creative work and present herself as an image of Aesthetic idealism, in essence synthesizing the subject/object split which had characterized the position of female viewers in relation to academic art throughout the nineteenth century. This assertion is possible only if one considers the act of Aesthetic dressing as a form of artistic production—a contested position which extends from critiques of the way in which design history and culture have marginalized and trivialized the making and wearing of clothing, and, more generally, fashion itself as valid art form.

As fashion was a socially sanctioned and even expected outlet for women's self-expression, Aesthetic dress was a logical outcropping of women's interest in artistic culture and design reform during the Victorian period. Various erudite and influential women served as examples of how women could carve out an artistic persona for themselves that re-sisted various normative cultural pressures. Perhaps the best example is the life and work of Marie Spartali Stillman, who was an active artist in Pre-Raphaelite circles. She both depicted Aesthetic themes in her paint-ing and wore Aesthetic dress as part of her artistic persona and produc-tion. Stillman was one of the more flamboyant and independent female artists who exhibited at the Grosvenor Gallery—an acknowledged center of Aesthetic culture during the 1880s. Sought after by many artists to sit for portraits and genre pieces, she was also prolific with her own art pro-duction and purposefully cultivated an Aestheticized image of herself. Her version of Aesthetic dress tended to adapt or reinvent styles of clothing as depicted in art; for the most part she utilized Renaissance portraits and Pre-Raphaelite imagery to inform her choices of attire. More than this, she repeated her own image in many of her works. Her image is inextri-cably linked with her own art and thus her role as a viewer and producer of art is synthetic and corporeal.[11] Wearing the clothes that she was often pictured in, her physical awareness of herself in Aesthetic dress may have been closely related to the images produced of her in Aesthetic raiment. This association reveals tension between representations of women in the visual culture of the Aesthetic movement and the embodied subjectivity of female artists, patrons, and viewers in those same artistic circles.[12]

The Aesthetic Tea Gown

As the most commercial and widespread instantiation of Aesthetic dress across a broader audience, the tea gown provides an excellent case study for teasing out some of the more complex intersections among Aestheti-cism, fashion, and imperialism. Several key elements of Aesthetic dress underpinned the rising visibility of the tea gown during the 1880s. One of the inherent contradictions of fashion, in general, is its ability to both reveal and conceal the identity of the wearer.[13] The dualism inherent in this relationship between artifice and deception on the one hand, and the revelation of the self through dress on the other, ultimately points to a romantic concern with an inner essence and sense of authenticity. This conception is articulated clearly in the debates surrounding artistic cul-ture and fashion. Utilized to search for a romantic ideal within oneself, Aesthetic dress proclaimed one's unique artistic sensibility, yet also func-tioned as an emblem of commonality—a sign that one was part of a larger group of individuals with advanced cultural knowledge. These dual func-tions informed the communication of Aesthetic tastes and preferences in the highly charged and gendered spaces of the nineteenth century, ranging from the private (tea time or the exhibition of one's collected art objects in the home) to the public (commercial and artistic exhibition spaces). Thus, as the ideology of separate spheres for men and women began to break down in the 1870s and 1880s, Aesthetic dress was an important factor in this process for many artistic women.

Evidence of a growing popular interest in Aesthetic dress can be found throughout the journal literature of the 1880s. Occasionally, visual illustrations accompany such articles, as was the case in *Queen* in 1881, where, despite the amusement caused by some expressions of Aesthetic culture, Aesthetic dress is noted as being "affected by many . . ." (figure 2.3).[14] Often, these descriptions point to the multifaceted nature of artistic dressing where the dominant references cover an eclectic mix of Orientalism, historicism, and neo-classicism. Especially during the early part of the 1880s, it is hard to pick up an issue of any of the leading British fashion journals without coming across at least one mention of Aesthetic dress. Although much of the fashion reportage is uniform and often repetitive, the detailed and descriptive use of language in some of the writing reveals an overriding interest in the ability of Aesthetic fashion to accommodate Victorian eclecticism and historicism:

Artistic dresses are on the increase. In the Row during the week many are seen, as, for example, a short dress of brocaded China silk of a grass green shade, the bodice pointed back and front . . . Old-gold finds many patrons among artistic dressers. With a short skirt of satin de Lyon and a long pointed piece coming from the back of the waist, a cream bodice and tunic of soft woollen material was worn, the sleeves puffed and tied between the puffings with bands of old-gold . . . An Indian red soft silk was made with a very wide Watteau plait at the back and a full banded bodice with tight sleeves . . . In the evening artistic dressing takes the form of a Watteau plait. A low square-bodiced dress of a tussore silk with one of these, worn at a dinner party last week, had the front gathered, but cut in one with the skirt, and not drawn in at all to the figure—a veritable smock.[15]

While rather vague with regard to its exact historical referents, such imagery is, nonetheless, artistic, flowery, and visually evocative, and serves to animate the text while invoking artistic discourses relevant to an art-savvy public. In this example the terminology used for Aesthetic gowns is significant; the origin of fabrics, both Asian and Indian, draws on the sumptuous exotic world of Orientalism and related discourses in the fine arts. "Old-gold," "satin de Lyon," slashed or banded sleeves, Watteau plaits extending from the back of the shoulders, and the references to smocking all recall fashionable details popular in earlier periods. The eclectic

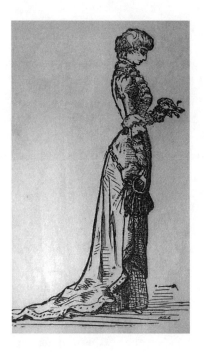

Figure 2.3 Aesthetic dress. *Queen*, vol. 69. (London. March 5, 1881). *Courtesy of the Toronto Public Library.*

combination of these various design details, and the luxurious savoring of language used to describe the ways in which these might be worn, point to historicism as an important facet of the antimodernism inherent in artistic dressing, and, further, firmly establish the link between artistic taste and colonial discourses of an exotic East.

Valerie Steele has argued that Aesthetic dress became more acceptable once it ceased to carry exclusive connotations to particular artistic communities or to the loose and immoral dress of neoclassicism. However, I would argue that it was precisely these earlier political and social connotations that popularized and drew interest toward the garments. In addition, Steele acknowledges that the fad for Aesthetic dress in the 1870s was ultimately "less significant than the more gradual adoption of artistic dress for private occasions in the wearer's home. The tea gown, for example, played an important role in the development of new styles of dress."[16] For scholars such as Steele, it was the gradual adoption and acceptance of garments like the tea gown into mainstream fashion that changed the popular perception of artistic dress and eventually encouraged widespread change in the fashion world during the first decades of the twentieth century. It is important to note that these new styles would not have been possible without the initial questioning of the accepted Victorian approaches to dressing. Further, this cultural shift hinged on an interest in the dress and clothing practices of other cultures, not only in terms of cut and construction (for example, the kimono) but also in terms of the ways in which alternate forms of clothing can serve as a form of sartorial critique accepted fashionable practices in the West (including the wearing of corsets and crinolines).

As artistically inspired tea gowns gradually became an acceptable way of dressing for fashionable women, the use of the tea gown expanded; often it would be worn at times other than teatime, particularly for hosting dinners at one's home. In the 1880 volume of *Cassell's Family Magazine*, a fashion commentator wrote: "Artistic dressing gains ground, and the Watteau style will be worn on many more occasions than last year. Tea-gowns have come to be the accepted style of dress for home dinner wear, and these are often made up with the Watteau plate."[17] By the 1890s, many fashion writers disagreed with the designation of "tea gown" for attire worn at dinner, due to the fact that many of these gowns differed little from fashionable eveningwear. One writer asserted that "tea gowns" were "unfairly called" as such, due to the fact that they were worn "principally at dinner-time."[18] Moreover, a growing level of anxiety and discomfort over the instability of the tea gown as a fashionable category was expressed in some of the journal literature of the time; writing for *Woman's World* in 1890, an author complained:

Life in the nineteenth century becomes more and more complex, and this is demonstrated as much as anything in the matter of dress . . . Now women dress for dinner in as many ways as the meal is served. Low gowns, half-high gowns, or tea-gowns which are akin to dressing-gowns, or tea-gowns that closely resemble the revised Court bodice inspired by the modes of mediaeval times— all these are popular, and you have to know the habits of your host and hostess when you pack your trunks for a round of visits.[19]

For many critics, wearing tea gowns outside the home was culturally inappropriate; the obverse side of this, of course, is that it can also be seen as subversive and disruptive of prescribed social roles for women. Just as the female shopper can be seen as an uncontrollable and unruly figure, the Aesthetic dresser, in a desire for innovation and experimentation, can be viewed as a destabilizing figure who cannot be controlled or contained by social roles and expectations.

The picture is not as simple as this, of course. While the increasing commercialization of Aestheticism can be viewed as positive or negative depending on your perspective, what cannot be disputed is the blurring of boundaries between public and private realms through an increased consumerism and the resulting reconstruction and transformation of gender roles. Susan Casteras has argued that Pre-Raphaelite approaches to the representation of feminine beauty, which started as a rejected and denigrated set of artistic principles, challenged Victorian canons of beauty and would eventually become the new standard for the pictorial representation of women in Victorian art.[20] While it is true that many forms of Aesthetic dress were derivative of Pre-Raphaelite ideals of beauty and naturalism, it is important to note that such ideals were often critical of mainstream values, and provided women with the means of questioning the constraints of a hegemonic and uniform understanding of femininity within Victorian culture. Further, as the meaning and representation of naturalism within Pre-Raphaelite art evolved, straying into the realm of decadence and symbolism, it can be argued that women artists, patrons, and viewers were increasingly aware of the discursive potential of "femininity" within Aestheticism as a set of highly constructed and fluid subjectivities and positions, and therefore open to alteration and intervention. Sartorial play, and the experimentation of fashion's boundaries within Aestheticism, in combination with consumer culture, can be viewed as enhancing women's experiences of, and participation in, the mechanisms of modernity in late nineteenth-century popular culture.

Stella Mary Newton has pointed out that dress, due to its perishable nature, responds quickly to changing social requirements and standards. The dress of the upper classes "has always responded more quickly than any of the other applied arts not only to changes in the social pattern but even to the first idealistic theories that have preceded them."[21] Such is the case with Aesthetic dress, which evolved in accordance with the changing sensibilities of Aesthetic practitioners. Yet the same currents that allowed dress to be acutely sensitive to the Aesthetic art scene also meant that such fashions were changeable, ephemeral, and inherently individual and eclectic. This is particularly true within Aestheticism, where subjective responses to art were emphasized rather than judgments of art based on social consensus or academic tradition. Aesthetic dress is a clear example of the negotiation between broader standards of taste within Aestheticism and the individual reception and exploration of embodied taste in practice. Although the emphasis on a purified Aesthetic realm over all other considerations can be seen to subvert normative class structures in Victorian culture, at least in principle, at the same time, it often called for the creation of a new aristocracy of taste: for example, James McNeill Whistler's self-professed oppositional stance as the artist-aesthete in opposition to the nouveau riche. However, it can be argued that Aesthetic dress allowed a measure of flexibility and social opportunity for those who wore it, although this formulation certainly excludes the poorest classes, who would have had little access or even exposure to Aesthetic modes of art and living. In her foundational text on nineteenth-century dress reform, Newton argued that the changeability of fashion was fertile ground for social protest and critique, and that rapid transformations in dress were the inevitable result.[22] Thus, I would argue that the complex relationship between standards of taste based on class groupings and Aesthetic preferences that partially obscured the distinctions of class-based fashion choices indicates the symbolic potential of Aesthetic dress to destabilize social norms and practices, not only in terms of gender but also in terms of class boundaries.

The Aesthetic tea gown was the first example of a wider dissemination of artistic dressing into mainstream fashion culture. At the same time, within the art spaces of the late nineteenth century, women's attendance and participation, as artists, viewers, and patrons, became more visible. Aesthetic dress was one of the ways in which women actively engaged with the artistic discourses of the day—gaining visibility and presence in a world traditionally dominated by male artists and patrons. As the practice of Aesthetic dressing gained momentum, it crossed the boundaries between traditional/conservative spaces such as the Royal Academy and alternative spaces like the Grosvenor Gallery. *Queen* regularly reported on the presence of Aesthetic dressers at the Grosvenor Private Views. In 1881 a reviewer wrote:

No wonder that the pictures on the walls occupy but the background of our thoughts; that the attention drifts away from them as our eyes rest on the face, it may be, of the painter whose hand has executed some of the most remarkable, or on that of an eminent poet, a grave philosopher, an actor or an actress whose personality is merged in our memory with that of ideal characters . . . The ladies' dresses showed last Friday at the Grosvenor Gallery that the aesthetic impulse is still active.[23]

In this quotation, the Aesthetic dresses worn are on equal footing with the activities and appearances of other "artistic" and notable personalities. There were those who publicly criticized the growing popularity of alternative forms of dress, viewing Aestheticism in dress as a movement against art and culture rather than as evidence of its democratic spread. W.P. Frith's depiction of Aesthetic dress being worn in his *Private View of the Royal Academy* (1881) illustrates the growing visibility of this style at semi-public artistic functions. The appearance of these gowns in otherwise fairly conservative artistic settings illustrates the ever-wider dispersal of Aesthetic dress. Although such examples are both within the realm of the art world, both the Grosvenor and the Royal Academy were highly visible public spaces. The presence of any kind of reform dress that questioned or contradicted the highly codified markers of mainstream fashionable dress during this time (tailored modest dresses, tightly corseted) would have been a reminder of women's expressive agency and their ability to physically embody their artistic preferences and proclivities. As a garment that gestured toward broader principles of dress reform, the Aesthetic tea gown was an important social and artistic cipher; both the wearing and artistic representation of such garments were ideologically and materially disruptive, offering creative ways to challenge mainstream Victorian sartorial norms and values.[24]

This breakdown or questioning of established Victorian social roles and spaces should be seen in relation to a more generalized fervor for design reform in the late nineteenth century. The trend toward improving taste in relation to Victorian lifestyles and spaces can be linked to the rise of liberal individualism and the newly acquired wealth mobilized by an emerging and influential middle class whose prosperity was based more on industry and commerce than on land ownership or inheritance. Diane Sachko Macleod has argued that the conflation of male and female roles of collector and interior designer within the Aesthetic movement coincided with increased leisure time for middle-class women interested in the arts, allowing them more time to "decipher the complex cultural codes of the Aesthetic movement."[25] Such intellectual and artistic machinations can ultimately be viewed as socially empowering for women. This is particularly true within Arts and Crafts circles, where modes of creative production typically gendered as "feminine" were not only valued but imitated and expropriated by male practitioners. Moreover, since subjective and reflective responses to art were valued highly within Aestheticism, this served to authenticate the experiences of female audiences, positioning them as participants in a broader Aesthetic culture, even if they themselves did not produce materially significant works of art.

Antimodernism and the Colonial Feminine

Self-expression, empowerment, and the ability of fashion to express simultaneously artifice and authenticity are central in a consideration of artistic dress as a catalyst for social change against the backdrop of modernity. However, it is also important to explore the degree to which the wearing of tea gowns was an extension of normative and regulatory social practices with regard to gender and race. Complicit in a larger field of colonial practices and attitudes, Victorian fashion can be examined for racializing themes that serve to maintain, and even enhance, dominant imperialist discourses of the period. The role of antimodernism in the perpetuation of cultural mythologies helps to explain the role of the tea gown as a significant and conflicted bearer of social meaning in Victorian culture. Aesthetic dress, dominated as it was by historical references and stylistic features, was symptomatic of a romantic withdrawal from certain aspects of modernity, most notably, the increasing homogeneity and mass culture resulting from ever-increasing levels of industrialization. One of the central features of antimodern images, texts, and writings is the use of pre-modern symbols to address the conditions of modernity. Paramount to antimodernist approaches to art and culture is the belief that authentic forms of experience—in the case of Aestheticism, an Aesthetic experience resulting from an encounter with the beautiful—will aid in the transformation of one's psyche in a recuperative way.[26]

However, with the growing emphasis on historicism, exoticism, and "foreign" goods across various retail settings, these "pre-modern" or "authentic" experiences threatened to be overtaken by the mechanisms of the modern marketplace. Leading design reformers and members of elite Aesthetic circles increasingly reacted against this commercialization of the art world and the sharp rise in the material consumption of Aesthetic lifestyles, goods, and services during the 1880s. T. J. Jackson Lears references this growing culture of consumption, arguing: "By exalting 'authentic' experience as an end in itself, antimodern impulses reinforced the shift from a Protestant ethos of salvation through self-denial to a therapeutic ideal of self-fulfillment in this world through exuberant health and intense experience."[27] Consumer spaces and mass-produced goods seemingly promised a type of "authentic" fulfillment for those audiences excluded from the higher echelons of Aestheticism. Although the method and means of absorbing and reflecting upon Aesthetic culture was often contested, the importance of consumer culture for female viewers and patrons, who may not have been artists themselves, reveals an important facet of Aestheticism's relationship to fashion, where widespread popular approaches were constantly being contested by the artistic expressions of a privileged few.

For those indulging in Aesthetic culture in commercialized settings, Liberty's was the destination of choice. Many fashion journalists praised Liberty's for their careful consideration and use of certain fabrics and manufacturing processes to maintain a high level of artistic quality and innovation, and, more importantly, a purportedly authentic relationship with Eastern sources. In an issue of *Queen* dated March 19, 1881, a fashion writer reported that the newest Mysore printed silks had been based on the "original wood blocks in the Indian Museum, of which exact reproductions have been produced. The silks are thin, and the designs and colours characteristic of their Eastern origin." A final seal of approval was given when the fashion writer concluded, "The aesthetic world will delight in them, and for dresses or upholstery . . . they would be suitable and uncommon."[28] The repetitive nature of advertisements, and journalistic reports on the latest fashions available at Liberty's, along with the favoring of Eastern, exotic, or archaic techniques in the production, dyeing, and finishing of fabrics for artistic dress or interior design, solidifies and centralizes Orientalist narratives in Victorian artistic culture. Thus, the link between consumer culture and Imperial conquest becomes inextricably bound up with the discourses of Aestheticism—particularly as it pertains to the decorative arts. Anne McClintock has argued that the allegiance between consumer spectacle and notions of a progressive Empire constitute a kind of "commodity racism."[29] However, since so much of Aestheticism is bound up in a sceptical or antimodern approach to art and culture, I believe that such spectacles within Aesthetic visual culture can be understood as both complicit with, and critical of, Imperial narratives of progress. On the one hand, visual representations of the "other," even when laudatory, serve to reinforce the notion of the West as distinct and progressive, and yet the exploration of, and positive attitudes toward, Eastern themes, images, artistic practices, and even materials, can also indicate a critical stance toward the traditions and regulatory mechanisms of Western culture.

An appropriate example and excellent case study for exploring the ways in which Orientalism informed discursive relationships between the modern and antimodern is presented in the work of James McNeill Whistler, who carried out several portraits of women wearing Aesthetic dress. One central work, wherein he designed and then painted an Aesthetic tea gown, actively engaged in colonial discourses and the visual culture of Orientalism. In his portrait of Frances Leyland, *Symphony in Flesh Colour and Pink*, 1871–1874 (figure 2.4), Whistler explored novel modes of artistic representation, reveling in a Baudelairean approach to fashion.[30] During the 1870s, the tea gown was similarly perceived as a novel form of dress, signaling the modern fashionability of a privileged subset of Victorian feminine culture. Its historical roots in the eighteenth century, as well as its romantic associations with specific medieval or Oriental themes within Aestheticism, were often buried within the intellectual and artistic writings of those deeply knowledgeable about Aestheticism. Whistler's work was generally considered experimental, modern, and innovative, which partially obscures and complicates a full understanding of the antimodern roots of Aesthetic culture. Whistler's modernist approach is an important structuring agent in his painterly preferences, and it is crucial to note that once Aesthetic dress became

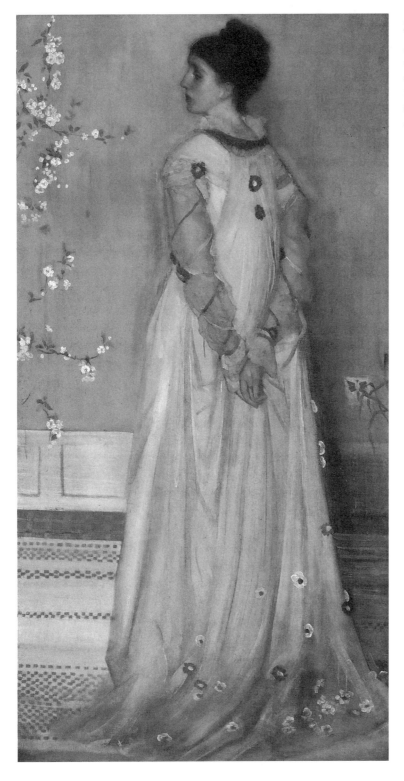

Figure 2.4 James McNeill
Whistler (1834–1903).
*Symphony in Flesh
Colour and Pink: Portrait
of Mrs. Frances Leyland.*
1871–1874. Oil on
canvas. *Courtesy of the
Frick Collection.* (Plate 3.)

more widespread and was no longer considered novel, Whistler lost interest in it and moved on to other forms of fashionable attire for his portraits. Yet his depiction of Frances Leyland in an Orientalizing tea gown represents an important moment when modern and antimodern themes within Aestheticism both determined the ways in which the Aesthetic female body was perceived and represented. Further, with its emphasis on individual and subjective artistic responses to visual culture, Aesthetic dress specifically, and Aestheticism more generally, was timely in providing a modern approach to past artistic ideals.

The tea gown pictured in *Symphony in Flesh Colour and Pink* is a hybrid of many competing and complementary stylistic features and traits. One of the clearest sources came from eighteenth-century fashionable dress, in the form of the Watteau plait. The dress also references the Japanese kimono, with the dropped neckline in the back connoting delicacy and sensuality. For many artistically inclined Europeans, the kimono also evoked the exotic elegance of the Japanese tea ceremony. Aileen Ribeiro has noted that, because of the comfort and elegance of the tea gown and its incorporation of historical and exotic influences, it became an "essential luxury" and a "garment of romance" that was inherently understood as both artistic *and* beautiful.[31] For Whistler, the tea gown's synthesis of Eastern and Western forms of elegance and beauty related directly to his own personal artistic outlook and approach, one that he most likely viewed as an original blend of Eastern and Western painterly influences and techniques. Margaret MacDonald has pointed out that many of his portraits represent a blend of Eastern and Western traditions.[32] Combining innovative painting approaches with thematic aspects of Orientalism and classicism, Whistler's desire to translate an authentic and intense artistic experience through the use of Eastern references and artistic techniques expresses fruitful tensions between the modern and the antimodern within Aestheticism.

This relationship is evident in Whistler's early work but is fully developed in his portrait of Frances Leyland. Susan Grace Galassi has argued that the dress in this portrait can be situated somewhere between earlier Pre-Raphaelite examples and later Aesthetic types, which it anticipates in some ways. Yet, she argues that, in its eclectic mix of historic features and current styles, it remains a unique creation that affirms Whistler's modernity.[33] Furthermore, I would argue that this dress in fact became a model for later Aesthetic gowns developing both in artistic circles and mainstream fashion throughout the following decade and until the early-to-mid 1880s. Deanna Bendix has even suggested that Whistler's delicate sensitivity to color, unified view of settings and interiors, and depiction of elegant figures all evoke the pose, costume, and coloring of a Watteau painting. She argues that the Rococo elegance, in combination with Eastern elements of Whistler's work, anticipates art nouveau figures and interiors of the 1890s.[34] In this way, it is in fact those very features of visual culture identified as antimodern—historicism and exoticism—that laid the groundwork for a "new" movement in the visual arts.

Whistler's interest in Japanese art becomes fully synthesized with his own aesthetic approach in this portrait. Certainly, Whistler was not alone in his interest in Orientalism and in realizing its importance for Aesthetic interiors. Paintings such as John Atkinson Grimshaw's *Dulce Domum* (1876–1885) and Edward Poynter's portrait *Lady Elcho* (1886) show Aesthetically dressed women in Aesthetic interiors, signified in large part by the presence of fans, blue and white china, and peacock feathers. However, there is a distinct difference between these examples and the work of Whistler. No longer connoted by obvious symbols or elements such as the use of blue-and-white china, the nature of Whistler's Orientalism is illustrated through his use of ambiguous spacing, the nuanced pose of the figure, and most importantly the presence of Aesthetic dress itself as the central theme and visual signifier. Branka Nakanishi has suggested that Whistler's pose for Frances Leyland may have found its origin in Japanese art. Some of the elements that point toward this conclusion are found earlier, in several of his "white girl" paintings; however, in this work, they have been fully developed and elaborated. The non-perspectival depiction of space, the decorative spray of flowers, and Whistler's butterfly monogram all evoke the appearance of Japanese prints. In addition, her pose may have been derived from Japanese woodblock prints; Ukiyo-e prints often pictured women from the rear in order to feature the backs of their kimonos as well as their necks.[35] The use of the Aesthetic tea gown to codify a range of diverse cultural references indicates the social function of fashion in expressing a complex range of interwoven cultural practices and artistic values.

It could be argued that, for Whistler, Aestheticism itself became a useful tool. The synthetic blending of Eastern influences, Orientalism and historicism, and his intense desire to express the novel, the original, and the artistically significant created for Whistler an abstract, aestheticized space of reflection, which referenced the modern world while at the same time allowing him to be removed from it. These contrasting tendencies in his work positioned him as a Baudelairean artist-dandy with a unique perspective on modernity, particularly within a British setting during the years between 1860 and 1880, when antimodernist themes were already well established in Pre-Raphaelite circles. It may even be said that

Aestheticism, as a swiftly changing and complex composite of artistic references and practices, served as a metaphor for Whistler's restless and ephemeral approach to painting. While Aestheticism privileged individual responses to art and indulged in the pleasures of viewing, so too did Whistler seem to value subjective and contingent responses to the visual. Aesthetic dress was an important facet of this experience; individual, eclectic, and ultimately subjective, it signified a level of sartorial distinction over and above the uniformity of mainstream fashion. Further, as an embodied social practice, Aesthetic dress may have stood for far more than social or artistic distinction, but may in fact have alluded to a shift from what was seen as visually pleasing to a more visceral form of aesthetic pleasure.

From a social-historical perspective, Whistler's work bore further significance in terms of its transformative effect on many Victorian artistic conventions. Ultimately, Aesthetic dress was emblematic of his developing artistic methodologies and his interest in modern modes of clothing for women in various art circles at that time. The visual congruity of Whistler's work and the artistic dress of female viewers and patrons is particularly notable since it is often referred to in the press of the day. During the famous trial between Whistler and Ruskin in 1878, a writer for *Mayfair* linked the erudite principles of high art with the fashions worn by the artistic crowd: "The ladies showed by their dress that they evidently knew more about the subject than the Judge, and when Mr. Whistler said that the knowledge which enabled him to knock off £200 worth of Thames landscape in a day or a forenoon was the result of a life's experience, the sentiment was received with loud applause."[36] Whistler's audience was vocal, present, and, most importantly, clearly identified by an outsider as "artistic." This marks the important impact of Whistler's artistic vision on his audience, and more significantly on the women involved in Aesthetic culture. Thus, Whistler's portrait of Leyland, and others like it, were reflections of how self-identified artistic women negotiated their artistic spaces and interiors, especially with regard to the wearing of tea gowns, which during the 1870s was the earliest sartorial expression of Aesthetic dress outside more elite artistic circles.

Accessing the views, experiences, and subjective responses of the wearers and consumers of Aesthetic dress provides a challenge. While multiple records of the perspectives of artists, writers, and critics exist, few accounts remain (or were likely undertaken) to translate and express the views of Aesthetic dressers themselves. We can, however, shed some light on the agency of Frances Leyland as a female sitter within Aesthetic culture; as both subject of the painting and agent of its creation, she is in a unique position, and, like many women pictured by male artists in the Aesthetic movement, her role in Aestheticism has been historically marginalized. Yet socially and ideologically, she played a crucial role in the dissemination of artistic principles. Leyland is one of the few sitters who claimed to have enjoyed the process of posing for Whistler. They became friends through the many sittings and there is clear evidence that they were close. Extant letters exchanged between them record the affection they felt for each other and the friendly accord they shared with regard to artistic issues. In a letter to Frances Leyland written sometime between 1868 and 1871, Whistler recorded his attempt to acquire some rare, artistic amber beads for her. He apparently sent them to her and enclosed a letter characterizing the beads as "the very best amber to be had at any price—beautiful in color and very pure . . ." Later in the letter, he refers to similar beads worn by one of the Spartali sisters, both well known for their beauty and artistic sensibility. He asserts: "It was quite a mistake of mine about the beads of Miss Spartali's being all equal in size—Lucas says they never are—and the effect would be clumsy and wrong on the neck—These are beautifully made—and will polish charmingly with an old silk handkerchief . . ."[37] It is clear that both Whistler and Frances Leyland were interested in fashion and artistic dress as a pursuit that might reflect their respective Aesthetic sensibilities, his as artist and hers as discerning patron. It is likely that in these exchanges Whistler's expertise allowed him to be an artistic guide or conduit through which Aesthetic culture was communicated. However, their relationship was not sharply asymmetrical, since Leyland's position as patron required a certain amount of deference on Whistler's part, and her decision to sit for him and continue an ongoing dialogue with him makes it clear that her interest in Aestheticism went beyond the superficial. The notion of self-fashioning was central in the artistic culture of Aestheticism.

Given that Orientalism was rampant in the visual culture of Victorian Britain, it played a crucial role in terms of the construction of gender and the possibilities, pleasures, and perils of the "female Aesthete." Through the lens of Orientalism and a post-colonial examination of the exoticism of tea gowns, one discovers that tea gowns in particular, and fashion more generally, complicate and magnify some of the debates surrounding gender, space, and identity in late nineteenth-century Britain. On the one hand, the feminine serves as "other" amid the standardization of male norms, preferences, and professions in Victorian Britain. Embodying the exotic roles of hostess, mistress, or model, particularly in domestic or privatized spaces associated with the feminine, women engaging in Aesthetic forms of dress reify concurrent notions of the "other" in the nineteenth century. A visual foil for masculinity as well as a foil for the body fashioned by Western standards of decorum, constraint, and modern fashionability, a British woman in "Eastern" or exotic dress symbolizes an overdetermined nexus of colonial and gendered discourses, which serve to position women in restrictive ways, both socially and ideologically.

At the same time, a British woman, particularly one in a privileged position with regard to social class, is definitively not a colonial subject, and in fact is an agent of imperialism, both in terms of race and class. Nevertheless, as I have argued, women who engaged in the practice of Aesthetic dress can be said to have participated in forms of meaningful cultural criticism, and ultimately were empowered in a creative and embodied way in part because intellectual freedom and play were enabled through the creative act of Aesthetic dressing. Playing with the codes of both fashion and culture, vacillating between masquerade and the sincere attempt to express one's inner essence, it can be argued that such women actively negotiated the complex terrain of social roles available to them. Ultimately, my argument rests on the assumption that an increased level of choice and intellectual mastery represents empowerment and social agency.

Fashion and the function of sartorial strategies in terms of cultural politics have been historically marginalized and/or trivialized. This fact alone means that often, particularly in the nineteenth century, women who engaged with culture on this level might have passed unnoticed, or might have been dismissed as non-threatening when compared with the more looming and pressing issues presented by activists, suffragettes, and other types of "New Women" who were actively questioning social norms in a confrontational way. In this context, however, fashion can be seen as a subversive field of cultural production—highly symbolic, central to identity formation, and yet largely disavowed as a cultural force of any import. Experimenting with the codes of fashion might have allowed Victorian women the relative freedom to envision and even put into practice principles, ideas, and strategies discouraged in more highly regimented areas of culture. Thus, ultimately, the practice of wearing Aesthetic tea gowns, which positioned women as both subjects and objects of a colonial gaze, could provide a crucial space for the negotiation of conflicting and competing social norms that would otherwise serve to marginalize or disempower women within the larger Victorian political and social sphere of normative and masculinized dominance and regulation. In turn, the discursive function of Orientalism is articulated in fascinating ways through the act of dressing oneself, and an analysis of fashion's seemingly irreverent use of cultural material allows us a unique glimpse into the complex and contested terrain of Victorian fashion where the binary distinction between constraint and freedom is no longer useful.

Notes

1. T.J. Jackson Lears has defined antimodernism as a critical engagement with the alienating aspects of modernity through a valorization of past or rural cultures and a perceived set of positive associations and social values. Lears, *No Place of Grace: Antimodernism and the Transformation of American Culture, 1880–1920* (New York: Pantheon Books, 1981), xiii.

2. In the realm of mainstream fashion, the tea gown was a garment deeply influenced by themes of antimodernism, due to its connection with Aestheticism and artistic modes of living. Prior to this commercialization of Aesthetic dress, artistic dressing was practiced primarily among cultural and artistic elites during the 1860s and 1870s. These included artists, patrons, and art audiences, who gathered at establishments such as the Grosvenor Gallery, and participated in the social circles and artistic events coalescing in the west part of London around the area of South Kensington. These styles tended to blend historical details from earlier British modes with more exotic features drawn from the arts and cultures of the Far East. Thus, while inspiring many contemporary portraits and modern genre pieces, Aesthetic dress was also heavily inflected by a growing interest in genre and literary paintings set in a distant or indeterminate past. Medievalism and classicism emerged along with Orientalism as the three predominant facets of Aesthetic dress in terms of its stylistic roots.

3. Reina Lewis, *Gendering Orientalism: Race, Femininity and Representation* (London: Routledge, 1996), 4.

4. An excellent overview of Aesthetic dress and its cultural significance is provided by Mary Blanchard in her chapter "Bohemian Bodies, the Female Body, and Aesthetic Dress," in *Oscar Wilde's America: Counterculture in the Gilded Age* (New Haven: Yale University Press, 1998). There are very few published books that adequately cover dress reform in the nineteenth century—even fewer that focus on Aesthetic or artistic forms of dress in a British context. Other than Blanchard's text, the only books that have focused on Aesthetic dress, in whole or in part, include Stella Mary Newton's *Health, Art & Reason: Dress Reformers of the 19th Century* (London: John Murray, 1974); Elizabeth Wilson's *Adorned in Dreams: Fashion and Modernity* (Berkeley: University of California Press, 1985); and, most recently, Patricia A. Cunningham's *Politics, Health, and Art: Reforming Women's Fashion, 1850–1920* (Kent, OH: Kent State University Press, 2003).

5. Regenia Gagnier, "Productive Bodies, Pleasured Bodies: On Victorian Aesthetics," in *Women and British Aestheticism*, ed. Talia Schaffer and Kathy Alexis Psomiades (Charlottesville and London: University Press of Virginia, 1999), 280.

6. Kathy Alexis Psomiades, "Beauty's Body: Gender Ideology and British Aestheticism," *Victorian Studies* 36 (Fall 1992): 32–33, 37, 48.

7. Erika Diane Rappaport, *Shopping for Pleasure: Women in the Making of London's West End* (Princeton: Princeton University Press, 2000), 6–12. Judith Walkowitz

has also explored the perceived impact of consumer culture on the subjectivity of female consumers in the nineteenth century, and further, has argued that the female shopper can be viewed as a destabilizing figure. See Judith R. Walkowitz, *City of Dreadful Delight: Narratives of Sexual Danger in Late-Victorian London* (Chicago: University of Chicago Press, 1992), 46–50. In addition to commercial spaces, political and social groups meeting for tea in the homes of women served to make private spaces more public. Such activities began to undo barriers that had previously contained and connected gender roles to specific types of spaces and practices. See also: Lynne Walker, "Home and Away: The Feminist Remapping of Public and Private Space in Victorian London," in *New Frontiers of Space, Bodies and Gender*, ed. Rosa Ainley (London: Routledge, 1998), 65–75.

8. Wilson, *Adorned in Dreams*, 144. See also: Elizabeth Wilson, "The Invisible Flâneur," in *Postmodern Cities and Spaces*, ed. Sophie Watson and Katherine Gibson (Oxford: Blackwell, 1995), 68.

9. Lynne Walker has suggested that the Arts and Crafts model and its celebration of typically feminine craft practices provided an alternate sphere for women in the arts, one that was relatively empowering for women when compared with the challenges they faced professionally in a wider artistic setting. Further, she notes that, by the end of the Arts and Crafts movement, there had been a significant increase in the number of women who functioned professionally as designers of their crafts rather than as executors of others' designs, proving that their involvement was increasing and significant even during the years they lacked adequate representation. See Lynne Walker, "The Arts and Crafts Alternative," in *A View from the Interior: Feminism, Women and Design*, ed. Judy Attfield and Pat Kirkham (London: Women's Press, 1988), 172.

10. Wilson, *Adorned in Dreams*, 9.

11. For a nuanced discussion on the significance of dress in the life and work of Marie Spartali Stillman, see: Deborah Cherry, *Painting Women: Victorian Women Artists* (London and New York: Routledge, 1993), 89–90; and Colleen Denney, *The Grosvenor Gallery: A Palace of Art in Victorian England* (New Haven: Yale Center for British Art, 1996), 160.

12. Alice Comyns Carr, in her published memoirs of her time among the bohemian elite in London's art scene, took great pains to note the dress and Aesthetic fashions of individuals such as Marie Spartali Stillman. In discussing the at-home parties given by the Burne-Jones family, she wrote: "The same people came Sunday after Sunday, and the party generally consisted of John Ruskin, George Howard (afterwards Earl of Carlisle), the beautiful Mrs. Stillman, who, though a painter of some note herself, often posed as Burne-Jones's model . . ." Alice Comyns Carr, *Mrs. J. Comyns Carr's Reminiscences*, ed. Eve Adam (London: Hutchinson & Co., 1926), 64.

13. Joanne Entwistle has emphasized the potential of fashion to articulate individualism while at the same time revealing a sense of commonality through its uniformity. In addition, in as much as dress is expressive of the self, it can also be used as a form of disguise or masquerade. Joanne Entwistle, *The Fashioned Body: Fashion, Dress and Modern Social Theory* (Cambridge, UK: Polity Press, 2000), 108–109.

14. *Queen* 69, March 5, 1881, 225.

15. "Dress and Fashion, London Fashions," *Queen* 68 (July 3, 1880): 7. "In the Row" likely refers to "Rotten Row," the fashionable thoroughfare in Hyde Park where people came to see and be seen during the London Season.

16. Valerie Steele, *Fashion and Eroticism: Ideals of Feminine Beauty from the Victorian Era to the Jazz Age* (New York: Oxford University Press, 1985), 157–58.

17. *Cassell's Family Magazine*, 1880, 441–42.

18. *Woman's World*, 1890, 25.

19. Mrs. Johnstone, "The Latest Fashions," *Woman's World* (1890): 75–76.

20. Susan Casteras, "Pre-Raphaelite Challenges to Victorian Canons of Beauty," in *The Pre-Raphaelites in Context* (San Marino, CA: Henry E. Huntington Library and Art Gallery, 1992), 19.

21. Stella Mary Newton, *Health, Art & Reason*, 2.

22. Newton, 2.

23. "Dress at the Private Views of the Grosvenor Gallery and the Royal Academy," *Queen* 69, January 8, 1881, 33.

24. While many "artistic" tea gowns were constructed along the lines of dress reform (intended to be worn without corsets, based on the principles of comfort and mobility, and the use of light breathable fabrics and/or vegetable-based dyes) it is important to note that Aesthetic details such as smocking were often used on more fashionably constructed tea gowns that were highly boned or intended to be worn with corsets and bustles. This appropriation of artistic discourses by mainstream fashion points to the hybrid nature of the tea gown, and its contested status during the 1880s as both fashionable *and* artistic.

25. Dianne Sachko Macleod, *Art and the Victorian Middle Class: Money and the Making of Cultural Identity* (Cambridge: Cambridge University Press, 1996), 289.

26. T. J. Lears notes that antimodernism was "not simply escapism; it was ambivalent, often coexisting with enthusiasm for material progress . . ." More importantly, Lears asserts that far from being the last nostalgic "flutterings" of a "dying Elite," antimodernism was a "complex blend of accommodation and protest which tells us a great deal about the beginnings of present-day values and attitudes." See Lears, xiii.

27. Lears, xiv.

28. *Queen* 69, March 19, 1881, 273.

29. Anne McClintock, *Imperial Leather: Race, Gender and Sexuality in the Colonial Contest* (London: Routledge, 1995), 33.

30. Baudelaire wrote that it is the business of the artist to "extract from fashion whatever element it may contain of poetry within history, to distill the eternal from the transitory." Further, he attacked historicism in fashion, stating that painters "though choosing subjects of a general nature and applicable to all ages, nevertheless persist in rigging them out in costumes of the Middle Ages, the Renaissance or the Orient." Typifying this response on the part of artists as "laziness" Baudelaire asserted that for many it seemed "much easier to decide outright that everything about the garb of an age is absolutely ugly than to devote oneself to the task of distilling from it the mysterious element of beauty that it may contain, however slight or minimal that element may be." Charles Baudelaire, *The Painter of Modern Life and Other Essays*, trans. Jonathan Mayne

(London: Phaidon, 1964), 12. This essay was originally published in installments in *Figaro*, November 26 and 28, and December 3, 1863.

31. Ribeiro mentions an early twentieth-century text that characterized tea gowns as "flowing garments of beauty," which drew associations among "a beautiful tea gown, daintily perfumed lingerie, and a love of art and beauty." Mrs. E. Pritchard, *The Cult of Chiffon* [London, 1902], quoted in Aileen Ribeiro, "Fashion and Whistler," in *Whistler, Women, & Fashion*, ed. Margaret F. MacDonald and others (New Haven and London: The Frick Collection in association with Yale University Press, 2003), 32.

32. Margaret F. MacDonald, "East and West: Sources and Influences," in *Whistler, Women & Fashion*, 67.

33. Susan Grace Galassi, "Whistler and Aesthetic Dress: Mrs. Frances Leyland," in *Whistler, Women & Fashion*, 95–96.

34. Deanna Bendix, *Diabolical Designs: Paintings, Interiors, and Exhibitions of James McNeill Whistler* (Washington and London: Smithsonian Press, 1995), 92.

35. Branka Nakanishi, "A Symphony Reexamined: An Unpublished Study for Whistler's Portrait of Mrs. Frances Leyland," *Museum Studies* 18, no. 2 (1992): 163.

36. *Mayfair*, Dec. 3, 1878 (Whistler PC2 Special Collections, University of Glasgow Library), 26.

37. J. M. Whistler in a letter to Frances Leyland, 1868–1871, Library of Congress (Manuscript Division, Pennell-Whistler Collection, PWC2/16/03), reprinted in *The Correspondence of James McNeill Whistler, 1855–1903*, ed. Margaret F. MacDonald, Patricia de Montfort, and Nigel Thorp, Online Centenary edition (Centre for Whistler Studies, University of Glasgow, 2003), at http://www.whistler.arts.gla.ac.uk/Correspondence.

Celia Marshik

❧ 3

SMART CLOTHES AT LOW PRICES

Alliances and Negotiations in the British Interwar Secondhand Clothing Trade

Advertisements for secondhand clothing dealers haunt the margins of British fashion periodicals of the 1920s and 1930s. Issues of *Vogue* and *Eve* report on the latest Paris models, but small notices remind contemporary readers that many women only came into contact with clothing designed by Chanel and Poiret—as well as with less august names—after other women had worn the garments and decided to sell them. Scholarship on fashion in modernity generally focuses on industrialization, mass production, and the rise of designer brands; Beverly Lemire speaks for many scholars when she asserts that secondhand apparel was only socially acceptable and widely worn before industrialization made cheaper, ready-made articles available.[1] Stanley Chapman, for his part, asserts that by 1860, eighty percent of the population of Britain purchased ready-made clothing.[2] Such arguments, which focus on the nineteenth century, occlude the ongoing demand for secondhand merchandise that persisted well into the twentieth century, a demand that indicates that preindustrial forms of the clothing trade quietly persisted at the edges of modernization.

This trade encouraged consumption of new clothing by underwriting additional purchases. As a 1932 *Vogue* "Shoppers and Buyers Guide" asserted, "here, when you are tired of your clothes and yet can't afford to give them away, is the name of a discreet firm who will buy them from you."[3] Through such advertisements, fashion magazines catered to—or at least recognized—that their readership comprised women of varying means.[4] These notices provide tantalizing glimpses of a trade in which upper-class, but not necessarily wealthy, individuals sold their clothing to women who were often further down the social scale with the assistance of a middlewoman. This trade required a complex negotiation of gender and class norms as both upper- and lower-class women needed the assistance of a woman in "trade" to make and maintain a fashionable modern appearance.

This essay provides new insight into the inner workings of the secondhand clothing trade by examining the records of Robina Wallis, who ran such a business by post between 1926 and 1959. The records of Wallis's business are now archived at the Victoria & Albert Museum's off-site storage facility, Blythe House.[5] It is difficult to ascertain how generalizable Wallis's business model is; as Lemire writes, the secondhand trade was "largely invisible" and left "few records."[6] It was clearly operated along different lines than urban secondhand shops, which often cultivated salon-style settings that, at their best, approximated the kinds of spaces where new clothing was sold.[7] Because of its very rarity, however, the Wallis archive is worth examining in some detail for the light it sheds both on the role of the secondhand trade in the "democratization" of dress and on the class, gender, and style norms that governed women's access to clothing.

Scholars of fashion and modernity have long debated whether fashion was "democratized" in the twentieth century—whether, in other words, fashion came within the realm of *all* consumers and not just the elite. Christopher Breward summarizes this thesis in *The Culture of Fashion*:

Britain between the wars has often been presented in terms of a sudden democratisation of fashionability due to advances in clothing technology, a further expansion of the publicity and advertising machine to incorporate film, radio and truly mass-circulation periodicals and a perceived broadening of employment and educational opportunities for women and the working class.[8]

As this account indicates, discussions of democratization have ignored the secondhand clothing trade, in part because it highlights continued disparities between privileged consumers and those with lower economic and social standing. By inserting the topic of the secondhand trade into this conversation, I suggest that the democratization thesis captures aspiration toward, rather than consumption of, interwar fashion. As I will argue, the Wallis archive demonstrates that even when women wanted to look "smart" and knew what that would require, the very fact that they negotiated deals with a trader like Wallis—and the types of deals they negotiated—serves as a reminder of the challenges many encountered when balancing their social and economic position with a desire for fashionable femininity.

The archive also demonstrates the peculiar form of intimacy established between the trader and her clients as the latter worked to maintain equilibrium between economy and appearance. Among other details, clients informed Wallis about their financial problems, social engagements, health, and general appearance when they corresponded about garments they might purchase. Such confidences were accompanied by a careful bargaining that demonstrates both shrewdness and a degree of privation on the part of buyers. The letters in the archive thus reveal that modern fashion mediated among women, creating complex relationships as well as barriers. Wallis's business provides an example of one of twentieth-century fashion's most enduring paradoxes: although mass culture created a widespread appetite for high style, clothing continued to magnify differences in purchasing power and personal appearance that remained stubbornly resistant to widespread change. When we think of twentieth-century fashion, then, we might most accurately see it as building a community that was not so much democratic as stratified even as it opened lines of communication among women of differing classes, conditions, and locations.

Robina Wallis's business was inherited from her mother, Mrs. E. M. Wallis, and originally operated out of Devon. The fact that two generations of Wallis women worked in the secondhand clothing trade mirrors the broader appeal of such businesses to women. As Chapman notes, nineteenth-century "slop shops" "were the easiest form of retail enterprise to start in the sense that the smallest amount of capital was required."[9] In addition, the trade appealed to women because, as Miles Lambert writes, "business could be conducted on a part-time basis, and in conjunction with another trade."[10] Such enterprises were also moveable, and at some point Robina Wallis herself relocated to Cornwall. After building her clientele through advertisements in *The Lady*, a weekly women's magazine, she sent and received garments from as far north as Scotland down to England's south coast. Wallis acquired clothing from society women, including the Duchess of Roxburghe and Lady Victor Paget, as well as from women in more modest circumstances. Some of Wallis's clients both bought and sold through her, suggesting that a number of garments made their way through multiple owners over time.

Wallis generally sent items on approval and issued credit to her customers. She kept careful ledgers that indicated how much she paid for garments, which items had been shipped to particular clients for inspection, and what was subsequently purchased or returned. Although her margin varied, she netted approximately £1 on larger-ticket items and three shillings on garments and accessories costing less than a pound. She circulated a variety of merchandise that spanned from humble corsets and gloves to more expensive items, such as a "brown cloth and beaver coat," which sold in 1926 for £25. Women wrote to her with specific requests for everything from mackintoshes to fashionable evening gowns. Occasionally, Wallis would also work with individual traders, who would try to find purchasers in their local communities. In 1936, for example, Wallis received a letter from Dorothy Eshelby, who wrote to return something she couldn't sell: "I cannot find anyone for the yellow costume so am returning it with the other things."[11] Working with women like Eshelby helped extend Wallis's reach and brought in new clients.

Businesses like Wallis's seem to have been a part of the national landscape, and the stigma associated with secondhand clothing—while never entirely absent[12]—lifted somewhat in light of the economic restrictions caused by the First World War and the Depression. During the war, a popular means of raising money for charity involved fairs or bazaars where working-class women could purchase designer gowns donated by society women.[13] And after the war, a class that came to be known as the "new poor" found that their prewar purchasing power would never return. *Queen*, a women's periodical aimed at the upper class, described this category as "those classes of education and refinement who have to meet the enormous increases in the cost of the barest necessities with steadily decreasing incomes, often enough on incomes reduced to the vanishing point by the loss of husband and father, or heavily encumbered, having the erstwhile breadwinner ill or disabled by wounds."[14] *The Lady*, in which Wallis advertised, exhorted its readers to adjust to such circumstances with good grace: "in these days of increasing expenditure and diminishing income, it behoves us—the new poor—to adapt ourselves to altered circumstances." The serial went on to praise the benefits of shedding "the last remnants of our false pride, our terror of 'what the neighbours will think.'"[15] Thus, while Lemire is correct to assert that "wearing cast-offs came to hold a stigma, to suggest poverty, and to smack of charity" toward the end of the nineteenth century,[16] worldwide conflicts and economic changes encouraged many British women to overcome their aversion to used clothing in the first half of the twentieth century.[17]

Novels of the period suggest that selling one's clothes was an expedient way for women in straitened circumstances to raise money. The narrator of E. M. Delafield's popular 1930 novel *Diary of a Provincial Lady*, for example, resolves to take this step as she ventures out for an elegant evening: "[f]inancial situation very low indeed, and must positively take steps to send assortment of old clothes to second-hand dealer for disposal. Am struck by false air of opulence with which I don fur coat, white gloves, and new shoes [...] and get into the car."[18] The narrator only receives a "rather inadequate Post Order" for her pains (141), but Delafield's novel—and the items in the Wallis archive—suggest that, in Peter Stallybrass's words, what little wealth such consumers possessed "was stored not [only] as *money* in *banks* but as *things* in the *house*."[19] Delafield's novel illustrates the ongoing appeal of selling secondhand clothing; in the 1930s, one's own garments were a source of quick cash.

Wallis's position as a woman selling clothes to other women was a distinct advantage in that it enabled her clients to share their love of dress with her, thus deepening customer loyalty. For example, a Mrs. Alderson Archer, who was evidently recovering from an illness, confessed, "I feel clothes are a bit of a nuisance when one isn't feeling well, but, if one gets just what one wants, it certainly does cheer one up."[20] This letter is something of a compliment to Wallis, who had the capacity to "cheer" her clients, and it also points to the emotional role clothing played in the exchanges between Wallis and her customers. Archer and others were not only interested in the price of the garments but hoped to get *exactly* what they wanted, a sentiment that indicates that clients did not want to compromise their standards when dealing with Wallis, even if they did so out of economic necessity. Other letters routinely contain thanks and appreciation for Wallis's work. Barbara Armstrong, for example, wrote not only to report what garments she would keep, but also to express her appreciation: "I have kept the grey tweed coat, it's such a nice one. Just what I want. [...] The black lace evening frock was most successful. Thank you so much."[21] Such letters no doubt helped Wallis's clients get additional items they would find suitable in the future; if the trader knew what individual women liked, it became easier to send them appropriate garments. At the same time, these letters cast Wallis as a female friend who brought happiness and pleasure through clothing: it is difficult to imagine that these missives would have contained such sentiments had they been addressed to a male trader. This gendered relationship no doubt helped to bridge the gap between Wallis and her clients, a gap not only of geographic distance but also of class and personal taste.

Although the documents in the Wallis archive indicate that women came together over a shared femininity and an emotional response to modern clothing, they also document the differences that femininity could not always bridge. Relationships between Wallis and her clients took place at a crossroads between intimacy and business; credit, debt, and differences of opinion rendered largely friendly bonds fragile. Letters in the archive demonstrate that clients were not only negotiating with Wallis but with modern fashion itself, and women's exchanges with the trader were complicated by a calculated sense of their social position as well as their financial wherewithal, which together rendered some styles and garments more desirable than others.

One site of conflict was the amount women came to owe Wallis. Her role as creditor enabled women to purchase items they might have otherwise returned, but it also created an obstacle to her trade when clients could not pay her. Ironically, at such moments women often shared the most intimate details of their lives with Wallis. For example, a G. Birch wrote on January 5, 1935, to ask, "with reference to my account—could you possibly grant me until end of March for settlement? My affairs will be in order [...] but the last few months I have not had my allowance to use having agreed to help some (Inlaws) over illness and other difficulties following on bereavement in their family."[22] The details of this letter serve to assure Wallis of future payment as Birch explains that her regular income is temporarily devoted to a different cause. At the same time, Birch's meticulous explanation sacrifices privacy—indeed, offers her privacy in exchange for extended credit—and provided Wallis with a glimpse of the private details of her client's life. Wallis probably never met Birch, but because she advanced the latter credit, she knew more about Birch's personal life and prospects than would be normal in a standard business relationship. It may have been Wallis's physical distance from her clients that made the sharing of such details possible. This is one of the very reasons that running a secondhand clothing business by post was beneficial to both clients and traders. If women couldn't go to a central shop and try on garments, they were assured of discretion and privacy because their patronage of such establishments—and their economic arrangements with the proprietor—could not be observed by friends and neighbors. And Wallis was not in a position to spread gossip about Birch as they lived in different parts of the country.

Although lower-middle- and working-class women were the most in need of Wallis's credit,[23] her business also put her in contact with evidently well-off women who similarly needed credit and patience and who shared intimate details of their lives with Wallis. In 1932, for example, Lesley Paul sent Wallis £4 but apologized for her inability to pay off her entire balance: "I would have sent the lot but the trustees are still quarreling as to whether my son (now 21) gets half the estate or not, so they are holding up my income."[24] Paul clearly came from a world of relative privilege, a world characterized by estates and trustees, but she still used Wallis's services and the credit the trader could extend. Clients evidently relied on Wallis's discretion and trusted she would not expose the fragile economic conditions they took pains to conceal with a fashionable wardrobe. As these kinds of letters (and Delafield's *Diary of a Provincial Lady*) demonstrate, a smart appearance often belied the financial troubles women experienced between the wars, and secondhand dealers could both mitigate (through purchase) and disguise (through extending credit) a woman's financial position. Wallis's business depended on her willingness to wait for a client's problems to sort themselves out as well as on her ability to calculate who was a worthy risk and who might never pay her. A client like Paul was clearly worth waiting for as her difficulties were temporary.

Sellers as well as buyers shared their economic woes with Wallis in letters that work both to exhort the trader to make money on their behalf as well as to promise more valuable goods in the future. In an unsigned letter from Paris dated February 22, 1927, one woman sent a plea for news as well as payment:

Having not heard from you about the fate of my last lot of clothes I wonder whether you have been able to do anything about them. I am rather badly in need of money and would be very pleased to get a cheque soon. Next month I will send you a navy blue coat trimmed with fur and hat to match, a crepe de chine dress and a skirt and jumper all in the same shade. Also a Chanel dress with a brown leather belt and brown felt hat. These articles are all good and I hope you will be able to sell them well.[25]

This seller had access to one of the most famous designers of the 1920s as well as to fine materials, but her letter to Wallis expresses economic struggles one might not expect a woman wearing Chanel to experience. Her plea demonstrates the important role that traders like Wallis played in the circulation of modern fashion; although many women who purchased designer clothing could afford to give away the garments when they tired of them, this letter writer made ends meet—and perhaps purchased new garments—with the funds she recouped by selling her clothing. The sale of these items put her in rather familiar contact with a woman she would not otherwise have known or socialized with, and she had to communicate her struggles to the trader at times. At the remove of Paris, the writer could share her condition quite openly as it became a means of pressing Wallis to sell her items for the best possible prices.

When Wallis couldn't get the prices her sellers wanted, they communicated their displeasure. Such moments posed a threat to Wallis's business; there were many secondhand clothing dealers operating during the period, and a dissatisfied seller might well take her items elsewhere in the future. In 1935, one woman wrote to complain about the return on her garments, expressing that she was "sorry you had let them go at half price as I would have had what I paid for them and that was 12/ for one set—that's what I paid and nowhere could anybody buy them at less price in the shops."[26] Although this seller did not couch her displeasure in terms of economic necessity, she felt that the market could bear a higher price than Wallis returned to her. It is unclear if the letter writer factored in Wallis's margin when considering her proceeds; any seller would make a greater profit through direct sales than through a broker like Wallis, and some women were willing to explore this option during the period.[27] Because this client appeared to expect that Wallis could charge the same price as "the shops," she does not seem to be particularly well versed in the value of items on the secondhand market. It is also possible that the seller saw the value of her items as a measure of her individual worth, and a low return thus became a kind of personal insult.[28] Such letters reveal that femininity could not always bridge the divide created by economic exchanges in which Wallis had comparative power over other women.

Economic necessity, then, motivated both buyers and sellers, leading them to use Wallis's services and to confide in someone who was all but a complete stranger. For the most part, women worked to cultivate the trader's favor in the interest of continuing the relationship, but disagreements arose when clients did not like the merchandise Wallis sent. While many women, like Mrs. Alderson Archer and Barbara Armstrong, were pleased with the garments they purchased through Wallis, letters that express dissatisfaction with what the trader dispatched provide a glimpse of what women expected from secondhand clothing and from Wallis in particular. Because Wallis needed to estimate which garments individual women would like, her skills as an interpreter of the needs of women she'd never met were always tested. If they didn't want items that Wallis sent for their inspection, buyers had to explain themselves in detail, sometimes confessing to physical and personal shortcomings or social limitations in order to justify their decisions.

Letters from Wallis's clients suggest that they expected they could get truly fashionable garments secondhand and not simply items in good condition. An A. Bailey, writing from Lower Hampshire, wrote to thank Wallis for a parcel but to reject some of the items it contained: "The jumper is not as smart as I wanted. I wonder if you have another one. I am sorry to give you so much trouble but I wanted a very nice one."[29] As this communication demonstrates, Bailey expected more than well-fitting garments—she wanted items that looked up-to-date and attractive. In such communications, it becomes clear that many clients refused to compromise their appearance even if they needed to purchase items secondhand; although Wallis's clients might have been "the new poor," their social aspirations were reflected in their desire to be fashionably dressed. Another client wrote from Devon to request a "smart black evening frock in either lace or georgette" and specified her desire for "a really good model."[30] Although Wallis's records do not indicate whether such women purchased exactly what they wanted, her clients obviously had access to some segment of the fashion press—which would inform them of what was "smart"—and used dealers like Wallis to assemble a wardrobe that bespoke a higher social and economic standing than they, in fact, occupied.

At the same time, some of Wallis's clients were aware that contemporary fashions did not always suit them and that their wardrobes must of necessity be more modest than those amassed by women fully in the fashion. G. Birch, the client whose payments to Wallis were held up by bereavement in her family, wrote on January 5, 1935, to return a fashionable accessory of the period: "Many thanks for so kindly sending the sequin coat. I am so sorry I cannot keep it as it is just a little too striking for me. Had it been a black sequin I could have worn it with most anything."[31] Birch's letter does not fully explain what made the coat "too striking" for her, but since she expresses a preference for a "black sequin" coat, it seems apparent that she needed garments that would coordinate with most of the items she owned and could not afford a coat that might be worn only occasionally. Clients like Birch wanted stylish garments, but their limited expenditures on dress meant that very fashionable and noticeable items were not wise purchases. In refusing the sequin coat, Birch demonstrated an awareness of her own social position and took intelligent charge of her wardrobe; far from a trivial choice, purchasing a garment required that Birch know and accurately place herself in a hierarchy of taste that made some "smart" garments inappropriate for her. In this case and others, the Wallis archives demonstrate that British women like Birch did not so much *consume* interwar fashion as *negotiate* it. As a result, the most desirable garments Wallis could send were contemporary styles that might "mix and match" with a variety of other items. Only in rare cases could a woman who patronized a trader like Wallis afford glitzy or unusual attire.[32]

Wallis's customers were also attentive to seasonably appropriate styles and used the fact that garments arrived out of season as a bargaining chip. Joan Donaldson wrote to ask Wallis to "reduce the two black dresses to £8 the two as the lace and organdie would have to go away until next summer. I like it very much indeed, but I seem to always be getting things that have to be put away."[33] Wallis's response to this letter was not preserved, and she might reasonably have refused Donaldson's request as more garments likely came her way out of season than in.[34] Donaldson's query suggests that buyers treated secondhand clothing as they would have items in the shops: dresses and other attire needed to be appropriate for the season in which they were purchased—an aspect of comfort but also of fashionability—and if garments were offered out of season, purchasers felt justified in asking for "sale" prices. Such letters indicate that many patrons did not expect to compromise their standards when purchasing secondhand clothing, and while such behavior might not have been entirely realistic in light of their economic position, the clientele for dealers like Wallis was not so much outside of the fashion system as trying to follow it as closely as possible while on a limited budget. Although the casual observer might assume that women who patronized the secondhand trade were driven by practicality rather than style, the Wallis archive makes clear that women did not view their consumption of used clothing as requiring a lowered degree of taste.

Given these standards, Wallis's clients also wanted garments that bore little evidence of their secondhand status. While some women seemed frustrated that stained or otherwise imperfect garments were perceived to be "good enough" for them, others used such condition as a means to bargain for a better price. In an undated letter, Lesley Paul wrote to return an ensemble because of its condition: "The coat and skirt is just rather well worn for what I want as I am invited to a very smart 'house party' in August. It includes some of my relations who would know at once that it was not new as they see me every day!"[35] Paul's letter indicates that women did not want to purchase garments that looked secondhand and, moreover, that they did not want their closest relations (those that saw them "every day") to know that they wore used clothing. For such women, secondhand clothing was only appealing if it looked new; as Paul's reference to the "smart 'house party'" suggests, some of Wallis's clientele moved in social circles aligned with a higher economic condition than they possessed, and "well worn" garments would reveal this disparity. This coat and skirt were accordingly returned.

Paul rejected garments that silently communicated their secondhand status, but an A. Linton, who wrote from Edinburgh, instead used condition to receive more favorable terms from Wallis. In an undated letter, she wrote that "the tweed suit fits well, but it has several large stains on the front of the skirt—perhaps you didn't notice them—I would give £3 for it."[36] The letter subtly upbraids Wallis, who should have noticed the stains and priced the garment accordingly, while it also works to achieve a better deal for Linton, who might have been able to remove the stains and thus purchase a tweed suit at a fraction of its original cost. This approach seems to have been routine for Linton; in another letter, she made an offer on a black gown that "wants cleaning and freshening." Such letters demonstrate that clients did not expect that garments Wallis sent would be marked by their previous owners. Some women, like Paul, would refuse these items outright, while others would use imperfections to bargain for a lower price. Comments on damaged or worn garments reveal their status as repositories of personal and group memory; indeed, as Stallybrass has written, "in the language of nineteenth century clothes-makers and repairers, the wrinkles in the elbow of a jacket or a sleeve were called 'memories.'" Although this charming word choice recasts a flaw as a nostalgic marker, Stallybrass notes that "every wrinkle or 'memory' was a devaluation of the commodity."[37] This was certainly true for Wallis's clientele, who wanted clothes *without* histories or memories. Both Paul and Linton's letters demonstrate that they are interested in much more than simple covering; their clothes needed to be blank slates on which the new owners could inscribe their own experiences. If *The Lady* was counseling its readers "to adapt ourselves to altered circumstances," such adaptation did not extend so far as to wearing garments that might give their secondhand status away.

Wallis's clients were also particular about their appearance in secondhand garments. M. A. Smith, who wrote to return a suit, was clearly not only concerned with cut, fit, and condition but also with whether a particular garment flattered her body type: "I am sorry to return enclosed, the suit fits nicely but the color is too light and makes me look so big. I was very disappointed. Maybe you will have something more suitable in a frock the next time you send."[38] Smith's letter identifies, explicitly and implicitly, two problems with her transaction. Smith's body was something of an obstacle to fashionability, but the letter also hints at Smith's disappointment with Wallis, who had sent something "unsuitable" for a woman of Smith's size and thus frustrated her client. Fashion columns of the day—such as Lady Duff Gordon's weekly article in the *Sunday Graphic*—emphasized which colors and cuts flattered different groups of women, and Smith evidently saw the import of color in selecting her garments. Smith, like other clients, was not desperate; she needed to buy used items to clothe an unfashionable body type, but she demanded that items she purchased look attractive on her. Wallis's patrons were thus economical *and* choosy.

When one reads the letters to Wallis and perceives the many reasons women returned garments to her—they weren't smart enough; they were too smart; they were out of season; they were worn or stained; the color wasn't flattering—it seems something of a wonder that any clients were completely satisfied by the clothing they purchased secondhand. But many women were repeat customers for years. For example, a Mrs. Yeoman bought items from Wallis between 1926 and 1941, a fifteen-year relationship that is unimaginable unless Yeoman's desires were satisfied by what Wallis supplied.[39] Wallis's business ledgers also itemize numerous garments that had a second life in her clients' closets, including a "black georgette evening dress" (sold to Lady Fairfax for £6), a "red crepe de chine dress" (Mrs. Smith; £5), a "Burberry Cape Coat" (Mrs. Symington; £3.10), and a "navy 'Poiret' dress" (Miss Donaldson; £5), among many other items.[40] The abundance and variety of merchandise Wallis traded speaks to the success of her business as well as to her skills in navigating the treacherous waters of economic limitations and the vagaries of personal style and appearance.

All of Wallis's skills, however, could not protect her business or her clients from the economic transformations that beset Britain during the first half of the twentieth century. If downturns and shortages made secondhand clothing appealing to some consumers, they also made such merchandise difficult to collect as time went on. After the British government began rationing clothes on June 1, 1941, civilians were encouraged to wear their old clothes instead of buying new. Oliver Lyttelton, President of the Board of Trade, advised his countrymen that "when you feel tired of your old clothes remember that by making them do you are contributing some part of an aeroplane, a gun or a tank."[41] In general, consumers were asked to "Make Do and Mend" during the war years, which reduced the circulation of used clothes.[42] In May of 1945, for example, an E. Baxter wrote Wallis an account of her troubles and promised to "send [Wallis] any clothes which come my way, only people are hanging on to them so."[43] The Second World War and the clothing shortages that came with it made secondhand items at once more desirable and harder to come by. Despite Baxter's difficulties and the general decrease in consumption of clothing during the war, Wallis managed to acquire some garments and continued her business through 1959.

The Robina Wallis archive illuminates the afterlives of modern fashion as garments moved from Paris and London to Lower Hampshire, Devon, and Edinburgh. These documents point to an important and unexamined component of twentieth-century fashion literacy and consumption habits, indicating that women were eager to purchase used clothing if it meant that they could buy a Burberry or Poiret garment instead of a new item from a less stylish maker. Sometimes clients received "just what one wants," and at such moments, it is tempting for a contemporary scholar to view the secondhand trade as truly liberating fashion for the "new poor." And yet, of course, many clients did not acquire precisely what they wanted through Wallis, or if they did so it was only by dint of patience, perseverance, and hard bargaining, not the leisurely consumption we tend to associate with modern fashion. In addition, their desires were themselves circumscribed by individual circumstances. Although Wallis's clients knew what was "smart" and might seek to obtain it, for example, in the case of a relatively inexpensive jumper, they recognized that some fashions were not appropriate for their social circle.

Wallis's business was just one of the many secondhand clothing businesses operating in Britain in the 1920s, 1930s, and 1940s. The January 7, 1925, issue of *The Queen: The Lady's Newspaper and Court Chronicle* advertised twelve such establishments; by May 2, 1928, British *Vogue* was advertising twenty-two secondhand dealers, and these numbers continued to climb throughout the year. Although such publications did not openly counsel readers to patronize these firms, their frequent gestures to economy suggest that many consumers would have found secondhand clothing appealing. The early July 1925 issue of *Vogue*, for example, included a "Seen at the Sales" column that explained why finding bargains was so important: "It is the aspiration of every class to imitate the habiliments and vices of the class immediately above it, and this is just what the Sale, magically, makes possible. It brings the unattainable (at all other seasons) within your reach."[44] This piece addressed what store discounts "made possible," but it also aptly describes the role of traders like Wallis, who offered women the opportunity to purchase the clothes "of the class immediately above" them and placed the otherwise "unattainable" in their wardrobe. At the same time, the *Vogue* column casts consumption of this type as imitation, a word that renders clothing bought at sales and through secondhand dealers as somehow inauthentic. As I hope I have shown, there was a distinct difference between the "new poor" and the comparatively well-off women whose garments they purchased, but imitation does not capture this relationship. Instead, we might most fruitfully think of the purchase of secondhand clothing as requiring *work* and, more importantly, *negotiation*, not only with a specific trader but with fashion itself. The letters in the Wallis archive amply document the complicated and sometimes difficult relationships spawned and sustained by this ongoing effort.

Modern fashion, then, was not only an expression of mass production and the ready-made. Although Lemire asserts that "[c]heap, fashionable clothing could be bought on every High Street in late nineteenth-century Britain," Breward provides the more accurate description of early twentieth-century fashion when he observes, "few even in the 1930s could afford the new clothes in the shops."[45] He concludes that "democratization" is thus an inappropriate characterization of British dress between the wars.[46] Although I concur that persistent differences in purchasing power made interwar fashion anything but democratic, the Wallis archive—and, one hopes, the archives of other secondhand clothing dealers yet to be unearthed from attics and closets around Britain—suggests that the used clothing trade went some way toward providing a wide range of women with access to otherwise unattainable garments. Such businesses also created cross-class communication that was characterized by a surprising intimacy as women worked, often successfully, to purchase "smart" clothing at low prices. Wallis's business didn't spread sartorial democracy, but it did offer discreet bargains year after year.

Notes

1. Beverly Lemire, "Consumerism in Preindustrial and Early Industrial England: The Trade in Secondhand Clothes," *The Journal of British Studies* 27 (1988): 21.

2. Stanley Chapman, "The Innovative Entrepreneurs in the British Ready-Made Clothing Industry," *Textile History* 24 (1993): 5.

3. "Shoppers and Buyers Guide," *Vogue*, January 6, 1932, 4.

4. British *Vogue* also sold its own patterns so readers could make their fashionable clothes at home. Sewing one's own clothes was yet another way women of limited means worked to look fashionable on a budget.

5. The archive contains letters written to Wallis by clients as well as ledgers of her business records. Unfortunately, Wallis's letters to her clients are not part of the collection.

6. Lemire, "Consumerism," 1.

7. For example, the early December 1923 issue of *Vogue* promoted a "Madame Longa" who claimed to operate "No shop. Just a comfortable salon" (109). Wallis's business was also distinct from a pawn shop in that clothes were sold, not pledged, through her, and she dealt in a higher quality of garment than was generally pawned.

8. Christopher Breward, *The Culture of Fashion* (Manchester: Manchester University Press, 1995), 199.

9. Chapman, "Innovative Entrepreneurs," 9. As Peter Stallybrass notes, during the nineteenth century, "not only did women do most of the pawning; it was their own clothes that they most commonly pawned to raise money for the household." See Peter Stallybrass, "Marx's Coat," in *Border Fetishisms: Material Objects in Unstable Spaces*, ed. Patricia Spyer (New York: Routledge, 1998), 204. Although pawning was distinct from selling clothes outright, both the buying and selling of secondhand garments had long been feminized by the time Wallis took over her mother's business.

10. Miles Lambert, "'Cast-off Wearing Apparell': The Consumption and Distribution of Secondhand Clothing in Northern England during the Long Eighteenth Century," *Textile History* 35 (2004): 14.

11. AAD/1989/8/1/104, Victoria & Albert Museum, Archive of Art and Design.

12. For example, one such business pledged to send "all correspondence under plain envelope." The promise of discretion indicates that it was somewhat shameful to sell or purchase let off clothes in the 1920s. See "Shoppers and Buyers Guide," *Vogue* (early July 1923): x.

13. See the "Page Mainly for Women," *Sunday Pictorial* (October 14, 1917): 10. Although the columnist asserts that "You would have laughed a few years ago at these girls [munitions workers] buying Paquin and Lucille gowns," she later concludes that "now—well, I think gowns should only be sold to women producing certification of war-work."

14. *Queen*, January 1920. Quoted in Breward, *Culture*, 201.

15. *The Lady*, June 24, 1920. Quoted in Breward, *Culture*, 202.

16. Lemire, "Consumerism," 23.

17. In the 1930s, even *Vogue* acknowledged a class of "the new poor" who could not afford to purchase many items in a season. Businesses like "The New Poor and Molly Strong Dress Agency" catered to "gentlewomen" who, like Wallis's customers, wanted secondhand items that didn't look secondhand. See "The Shoppers' and Buyers' Guide," *Vogue*, January 6, 1932, 4.

18. E. M. Delafield, *Diary of a Provincial Lady* (Chicago: Academy of Chicago, 2002), 118. Further references cited in the text. The narrator later reports that she collected the "major portion of my wardrobe and dispatch to address mentioned in advertisement pages of *Time and Tide* as prepared to pay Highest Prices for Outworn Garments" (138). This fictional event underlines the role of advertising in building up secondhand businesses that operated by post as well as the importance sellers placed on promises of high returns.

19. Stallybrass, "Marx's Coat," 202.

20. AAD/1989/8/1/2, Victoria & Albert Museum, Archive of Art and Design. Archer's letter is dated March 26.

21. AAD/1989/8/1/5, Victoria & Albert Museum, Archive of Art and Design. Armstrong's letter is dated June 28.

22. AAD/1989/8/1/24, Victoria & Albert Museum, Archive of Art and Design.

23. For example, in November 1932, a Mabel E. Long wrote to apologize for her delinquency: "Things mount up so quickly and I have not received some money I hoped to have. Everything is paying so badly." Long was still behind on her payments in 1934 (AAD/1989/8/1/124, Victoria & Albert Museum, Archive of Art and Design).

24. AAD1989/8/1/153, Victoria & Albert Museum, Archive of Art and Design.

25. This letter was tucked into Wallis's ledger of accounts with sellers (AAD/1989/8/3/1) and does not have a catalog number.

26. AAD/1989/8/1/169, Victoria & Albert Museum, Archive of Art and Design.

27. For example, in the 1920s *The Gentlewoman in Town and Country* operated "The 'G' Private Exchange." Every subscriber could place a short advertisement each week for garments, household items, or other things. *The Gentlewoman* even

ran a kind of bank so subscribers could inspect the goods; if one wanted to buy, one sent the G. the amount and the paper had the seller send the item. If it wasn't returned, the G. paid the seller. This arrangement removed the middle-woman from the exchange and thus insured higher prices, but sellers had to sacrifice some of their privacy in dealing directly with would-be purchasers.

28. This dynamic is evident in Delafield's novel, wherein the provincial lady is shocked to find that only "three-and-sixpence" is being charged for "grey georgette only sacrificed [to a local charity's Jumble Sale] at eleventh hour from my wardrobe" (241).

29. AAD/1989/8/1/15, Victoria & Albert Museum, Archive of Art and Design. Bailey's letter is undated.

30. AAD/1989/8/1/7, Victoria & Albert Museum, Archive of Art and Design. The letter is undated.

31. AAD/1989/8/1/24, Victoria & Albert Museum, Archive of Art and Design.

32. For this very reason, the secondhand dealer in Delafield's novel returns as "unsaleable" a "white tennis coat trimmed with rabbit" (141). Such a striking garment was simply not the kind of thing most women could afford to buy, even secondhand.

33. AAD/1989/8/1/88, Victoria & Albert Museum, Archive of Art and Design. The letter is undated.

34. Most women sold clothing at the end, not the beginning, of the season. An exception is Mrs. William Phipps, who wrote to say she was sending "5 summer dresses—they are all in perfect condition and very little worn but I shall not be in the country so think I had better sell them." (AAD/1989/8/1/156, Victoria & Albert Museum, Archive of Art and Design. No date).

35. AAD 1989/8/1/155, Victoria & Albert Museum, Archive of Art and Design.

36. AAD/ 1989/8/1/122, Victoria & Albert Museum, Archive of Art and Design.

37. Stallybrass, "Marx's Coat," 196.

38. AAD/1989/8/1/168, Victoria & Albert Museum, Archive of Art and Design. Smith's letter is undated.

39. Yeoman's contact with Wallis is documented in a ledger (AAD/1989/8/3/2, Victoria & Albert Museum, Archive of Art and Design) that only covers 1926–1941. Because Wallis remained in business through 1959, it is possible that Yeoman was a client for even longer.

40. These garments are among the many itemized in Wallis's sales ledger (AAD/1989/8/3/2, Victoria & Albert Museum, Archive of Art and Design).

41. Quoted in Monica Charlot, *British Civilians in the Second World War* (Paris: Didier Érudition, 1996): 95.

42. Ibid., 98.

43. AAD/1989/8/1/23, Victoria & Albert Museum, Archive of Art and Design.

44. "Seen at the Sales," *Vogue*, early July 1925, 33.

45. Lemire, "Consumerism," 22; and Breward, *Culture*, 187.

46. Breward, *Culture*, 199.

II

FASHION AND CULTURAL ANXIETY

Ellen Bayuk Rosenman

❦ 4

FEAR OF FASHION; OR, HOW THE COQUETTE GOT HER BAD NAME

Victorian culture perfected a fashion double bind that is still with us today: women are required to invest themselves deeply in their appearance and then derided for this obsession.[1] On the one hand, dressing well was declared to be women's "duty," their contribution to the pleasures of society.[2] Yet at the same time, a woman who took this duty too seriously, or discharged it too successfully, was charged with vanity—or "VANITY," as one commentator puts it, to register his outrage typographically in no uncertain terms.[3]

Why was this double bind necessary? Behind the trivialization of fashion lie anxieties about what women are actually doing in the social zones designated for their marginalization, left dangerously unpoliced by men. At the center of these anxieties stands the coquette, that ubiquitous figure on the Victorian landscape, demonized, I argue, because she represents forms of agency and desire that threaten social norms. She is well known as a seductress, but her sexual power—alarming but nonetheless part of traditional ideas about femininity—is only part of her significance. The coquette raises fears because of her expertise as well as her allure, because of her passion for clothing for its own sake as well as her desire to captivate men. For while fashion is generally understood as a kind of female ghetto, it often functioned as a liminal area that jeopardized gender distinctions and the heterosexual imperative.

While attacks on female vanity certainly predate the Victorian era, new developments in commerce and print culture intensified and in some ways refocused the energies and anxieties of fashion critics, as a number of scholars have argued. By the mid-nineteenth century, fashion had simultaneously become democratized and commercialized: more and more articles of clothing were available in shops, especially in urban areas. Shopping was transformed, redefined in terms of leisure and pleasure rather than utilitarian acquisition. Building on the practices of specialized "large-scale and fast-selling" eighteenth-century stores, Victorian shops expanded both their inventory and their marketing techniques.[4] Quiet interiors blossomed into gorgeous showrooms. Newly developed in the 1830s and widely used by the 1850s, plate-glass windows framed carefully designed displays, further aestheticizing fashion, while gas lighting burnished goods with an enticing glow. Eager to draw female customers, high-end stores simulated the comforts of home, providing luxurious lounges in which women could recover from the arduous business of consumption and fortify themselves with refreshments. In Erika Rappaport's memorable phrase, the Victorian era invented "shopping for pleasure."[5]

At the same time, a burgeoning print culture made shopping, clothing, and fashion matters of public concern. Fueled by developments in paper-making, transportation, and the mechanical reproduction of texts, the periodical press disseminated cultural issues, conflicts, and anxieties more widely than ever before. In the words of Laurel Brake and Julie Codell, "as the site of debates and encounters, the press emerged as a major public space for discourses about society, politics, [and] culture."[6] Women's magazines played a special, though far from exclusive, role in this discussion. With enhanced production values made possible by technological advances, a new generation of women's magazines circulated images of beautiful women, presented the latest fashions, and offered beauty advice, tacitly asserting that "fashion was a necessary ingredient" in women's reading and their lives.[7] While men continued to concern themselves with the impression made by their clothing, their styles became more subtle as Regency flamboyance died out—a development that seemed to imply that women were invested in their appearance with a gender-specific narcissism.[8]

In this rich material and discursive moment, fashion emerged as a battleground between the sexes. On the one side, coquettes allegedly plundered fashionable shops for modish clothing to attract male attention, creating the illusion of natural grace and beauty. On the other, men strove to learn these devices, see through the false exterior, and arm themselves against a seduction that might lead to a miserable liaison, or even to marriage, with a lower-class, depraved, or otherwise unworthy woman. Thus Alexander Walker, amateur philosopher and physiologist, attempts to demystify women's beauty secrets in his popular work *Beauty in Woman Analysed and Classified with a Critical View of the Hypotheses of the Most Eminent Writers, Painters, and Sculptors*.[9] For all his apocalyptic warnings about women's sexual allure, Walker seems equally concerned about the knowledge-power wielded by the coquette, whose seduction depends on an intimate knowledge of fashion and its aesthetic effects. To counter such knowledge, Walker draws extensively on philosophers such as Hogarth and Hume in order to examine women's beauty from within a purportedly objective, rational framework. He attempts to demystify women's seductive beauty most strenuously in a chapter entitled "External Indications; or the Art of Determining the Precise Figure, the Degree of Beauty, the Mind, the Habits, and the Age of Women, notwithstanding the Aids and Disguises of Dress." After teaching men how to observe a woman's posture and gait to determine her health and "conformation," Walker cautions, "Even with regard to the parts of the figure which are more exposed to observation by the closer adaptation of dress, much deception occurs. It is, therefore, necessary to understand the arts employed for this purpose, at least by skilful women" (330, 331). Describing bonnet styles that flatter particular faces, clothing that enhances taller or shorter women, and colors that improve problem complexions, he admonishes men to pay special attention to the linings of bonnets, which are especially well positioned to lend the face an unfair advantage. Ever the manipulator, the skilful woman deliberately conceals them: "care is . . . taken that these linings do not come into direct view of the observer" (Walker, 335). Walker even urges men to analyze the decor of women's homes, since "apartments may, indeed, be peculiarly calculated to improve individual complexions" (336).

Walker assures men that this knowledge is well within their reach: "in society we every day hear women pronounce perfectly correct opinions as to the proportions of the neck, the bosom, the hands, and the arms of other women . . . If so, it is certainly in the power of a man of science, with as observing an eye, to go still further, and conceive many other necessary circumstances concerning proportion" (254). But despite the assurance that the man of science can boldly go where no woman has gone before, this passage reflects the recognition that women have already pioneered the techniques that men must now struggle to decode. The aesthetic principles were discussed in the new fashion magazines of the period such as *The Ladies' Pocket Magazine*, which presented nearly identical information to Walker's external indications in an article entitled "Colours for Female Dress." Giving examples of colors that flatter different complexions (though not going so far as to suggest interior decorating schemes), the article concludes, "The elementary truths [of color combinations] may form the ground-work of further reflection"— exactly the kind of cogitation Walker fears.[10] The proliferation of these femininity manuals created the image of a female culture that men would disdain, Walker implies, at their peril. Furthermore, this *kind* of knowledge—concrete, practical, social—contests the authority of Walker's abstract philosophical axioms. "Goodness and beauty in woman will accordingly be found to bear a strict relation to each other; and the latter will be seen always to be the external sign of the former," Walker assures the reader (27). But, as his treatise acknowledges, women's mastery in the realm of the everyday, so often gendered feminine and devalued, can overcome the body's putative transparency.[11] In this light, it is possible to regard Walker's endless quotations of philosophers as an elaborate ruse to disguise the fact that the truly salient knowledge lies, not in the theories of Hume and Hogarth, but in women's culture. His condemnation of the coquette derives at least in part from the fear of this potent if unofficial expertise to which women have the superior claim.

Ironically, then, although fashion presents itself as a signifier of gender identity, both because clothes distinguish men from women and because interest in clothes is typed as feminine, it also tends to collapse a gender hierarchy based on knowledge and expertise. Analyzing the practices of the coquette within the context of legitimate aesthetics, Walker comes dangerously close to acknowledging fashion as an art form, as women themselves sometimes asserted. In the deliberately titled *The Art of Beauty and the Art of Dress*, Eliza Haweis explicitly links fashion and art, declaring "what is true in painting is also true in dress" and identifying museums as sources of fashion inspiration.[12] And while this connection did not endow well-dressed women with the same cultural capital as painters or writers, it does present a plausible view of fashion's cultural place.[13] By raiding the visual arts for new ideas, Victorian fashion repeatedly traversed the boundary between high culture and inferior arenas. As fashion historians argue, aristocratic portraits were primary purveyors of fashion knowledge.[14] Far from remaining safely entrenched in manor houses and museums as tokens of upper-class privilege, they reappeared in fashion plates. Easily removed from the magazine and suitable for framing, these illustrations were skillfully and artistically rendered: the same *Ladies' Pocket Magazine* that offered advice about colors also assured its readers that "the Engravings will continue to be furnished by eminent artists, from pleasing and interesting designs by the most eminent masters of the British and Foreign Schools of Painting," adding that their fashion plates would henceforth be made with steel rather than inferior copper plates ("Preface" 60). Many illustrations presented models in contemporary dress, while others posed women in classical settings and styles.[15] Others circulated images of aristocratic beauties, offering readers a cut-rate, accessible version of the family paintings hung in manor homes. The portrait of Lady Dedlock in *Bleak House* is representative: displayed for admiring strangers who visit the Dedlock estate like reverent museum-goers and described as "the best work of the master" by a helpful housemaid-docent, it reaches a wider audience in the fictitious *Galaxy of Beauties*, modeled on a host of real-life fashion magazines.[16] In her witty juxtaposition of Blake engravings and contemporary illustrations of women's clothing, which she calls "biblical fashion plates," Anne Hollander asserts a continuity between high art and fashion: the images are almost identical despite the difference in purpose, suggesting the ease with which high art could be appropriated and recontextualized.[17] Recognizing the potential of this appropriation, Charles Frederick Worth, the father of haute couture, developed his storehouse of ideas by wandering London's National Portrait Gallery in the 1840s.

In short, fashion bled dangerously into more respectable and less feminine forms of knowledge, suggesting that women possessed an expertise that was not only sexually dangerous but bespoke a sophisticated sense of line, form, and color that could only be termed "artistic." Walker's strategy of reappropriation was not uncommon; increasingly, clothing was dealt with as a serious intellectual matter under male jurisdiction. It was colonized in a spate of historical and anthropological analyses in the periodical press that removed fashion from its immediate social and sexual context. A typical example is "Beautiful For Ever," which surveyed the history of beauty from "the first toilet[te]" through the Greeks and Romans, and on to the present day.[18] In its early years, *Cornhill Magazine* showed particular interest in the subject of fashion, featuring several essays in its first years of publication: "Paint, Powder, Patches" reports on the beautification customs of the Orient, the ancient Europeans, the Hottentots, and the Transatlantic Indians; "Costume and Character" surveys the dress of the Spanish, Turks, Greeks, Armenians, and Arabs; "Good Looks" presents anecdotes about Tamerlane's wife, Cicero, Queen Elizabeth, and an African chief visiting England. In this welter of expert information, fashion as a site of struggle between the sexes becomes neutralized as the subject of dispassionate scholarly inquiry, and women's expertise is crowded out of the picture. Indeed, history could be used to chastise women for their aesthetic pretensions: "the great artists and the great conquerors of the world never tolerated any thing beyond this flowing drapery of the veil," one writer declares, surveying women's headdresses through the ages to expose the absurdity of contemporary styles.[19]

Like popular history and anthropology, physiology was also deployed to contest female authority, asserting the primacy of scientific knowledge over the claims of fashion practitioners. Once the province of moralists, attacks on female vanity could be reworked in the emerging professional discourse of scientific medicine, lending them a new air of objectivity.[20] While objections to tight lacing responded to genuine physical risks, other attacks seem more concerned with establishing control over women's bodily self-management.[21] Seeking to establish the proper authority of doctors and to correct "the follies of fashion" with a medical view of the human body, one article lamented, "M. Worth, for instance, is far more powerful, as things are, than the College of Physicians; and the fiats of a fashionable bootmaker or corset manufacturer are supreme, when compared with the expostulations of the physiologist."[22] No less a public intellectual than George Henry Lewes lectured women about their "blank ignorance" regarding the human body: "if you knew how your skin was constructed, how it grew and breathed, and how it assumed its 'complexion,' you would as soon think of remedying its defects by the use of cosmetics, as of rendering hieroglyphics legible by whitewashing a monument."[23] Doctors themselves entered the arena, delivering their professional opinions in general-interest periodicals. Passing judgment on the evening dress, one J. Milner Fothergill, MD, declared that "Physiology says such dresses are a violation of the laws of health," along with heeled shoes and flimsy bonnets.[24] Popular works such as Erasmus Wilson's *Healthy Skin: A Popular Treatise on the Skin and Hair, Their Preservation and Management* and Arnold J. Cooley's *The Toilet and Cosmetic Arts in Ancient and Modern Times* furthered such arguments. The latter combined the historical, philosophical, and scientific approaches: it surveyed the use of cosmetics from the Greeks, appealed to the wisdom of Hume and Burke like Walker's *Beauty in Woman*, and concluded with chemical formulas for health and beauty aids. Such texts assert that science, history, and anthropology—not fashion magazines—will provide the authorized version of the female body.

Alongside these discursive battles over the status of fashion and fashion knowledge, the selling and buying of women's clothes further upset the gender hierarchy by generating new social actors, relationships, and forms of erotic experience. "Window dressers"—young women who modeled the wares of clothing stores—and the shopgirls who sold the merchandise displayed themselves, earned money, and developed a notoriously flirtatious boldness through their work, turning a stereotypically feminine interest in clothing into a public and remunerative enterprise.[25] Often they stood at the doorway of the store to lure in indecisive pedestrians, as if signaling their position at the threshold of the public world of commerce.[26] Masculinity, too, was compromised in this woman-identified world. Young men employed by women's clothing stores to arrange window displays and assist customers seemed to catch femininity through their occupations as if it were a contagious disease. The *Morning Chronicle* describes the desexing of one such degraded creature employed by a millinery shop:

> A soft automaton in shape of man,
> Powder'd and perfum'd, see the creature stalk,
> Smirk like a lady, delicately talk,
> Choose out a headdress, praise lace stuffs[27]

Even more alarming was the male milliner. While the shop-boy described above could simply be satirized as effeminate and dismissed, the male milliner was more difficult to categorize. A hybrid figure, he shared the fashion expertise of women but remained a respectable and successful businessman. After reporting with mock astonishment that "there are bearded milliners ... milliners in pantaloons" presiding over city shops, *All the Year Round* goes on to call them "authentic men" and to rehabilitate their suspect manhood: "There is not the slightest intention here to cast disfavour on the talent of the English artist, and still less on his personal character; he has a profession which he exercises. He is engaged in a commercial undertaking."[28] Veering between sarcasm and seriousness, the tone of the article betrays the gender confusion provoked by this figure. Nothing could be more respectably male than to "engage in a commercial undertaking," nothing more feminine than to display a deep investment in a well-cut frock.

But perhaps most disturbing was a new breed of female shopper, who discovered that "shopping for pleasure" could rival, and even surpass, the rewards of heterosexuality. Fashion historian C. Willett Cunnington reports a comic incident in which a father is about to attack a man who appears to be embracing his young daughter, only to discover that the man is fitting her with "bosom friends"—that is, wax falsies.[29] This is the most suspect pleasure of fashion, that it is not a heterosexual encounter but the autoerotic delight of bodily self-cultivation.[30] Behind the snobbish dismissal of women and their milliners, male or female, lies a suspicion about the secret goings-on in the boudoir and the shop, to which masculine men—that is, men who do not share this passion for fashion— are superfluous. If the traditional coquette of novels and conduct books threatens men with seduction, another version of the coquette threatens them with something far worse—indifference. In the custom of consulting a famous designer before making an appearance at a ball, the clothing salon appears as a parallel universe to the world of courtship, complete with its own nearly identical delights. Elegant women arrive at the shop in their carriages, partake of a delicious buffet, display their finery—in short, they do everything they will do at a ball except dance with men.[31] It is only a step from this parallel universe to the ultimate self-sufficiency: a woman's relationship to her own body and image. Frequently evoked with the emblem of the mirror—as when Gwendolen Harleth in *Daniel Deronda* kisses her beautiful reflection like a Victorian Narcissus—the self-absorption of the coquette is a further threat to heterosexuality.[32]

The same article that puzzles over male milliners presents the poignant story of a rich man married to such a narcissist. As she models each new and expensive outfit for his approval, he thinks with delight about how much she wants to please him. But when he receives several bills far beyond her clothing allowance and forbids her to buy anything more, she sulks and pines. What she loves is not him but clothing and her own image. While the article presents itself as a cautionary tale about the wages of female vanity, it might also be read against the grain as a tale about *male* narcissism, in the husband's assumption that his wife's efforts exist to gratify him. To quote Baudrillard's gloss on seduction, this husband has read into his wife's self-presentation a flattering if deluded message about his own priority, as if she were a traditional coquette bent on attracting his admiration: "I am attractive, but you are captivating."[33] In reality, as he discovers, his wife is a separate subject who lives in a world with its own values and concerns, which he has failed to even imagine. He is stunned not only by his wife's extravagance but by her deep investment in fashion for its own sake, in contrast to her tenuous and instrumental investment in him. While the story assumes that clothing is trivial and the wife's fetish simply announces her shallowness, we can also read it as the tale of an unappreciated artist, as the wife presents outfit after delectable outfit to her obtuse husband, who can only muster a single word of praise on each occasion ("Perfect!") and ponder the depth of his wife's adoration. For the skilful woman, fashion may be, as Anne Hollander suggests, a legitimate "visual art" and the narcissistic mirror-gazing a form of self-portraiture, one whose audience is the woman herself and not a philistine husband who must consult a treatise like Walker's *Beauty in Woman* to recognize an artful bonnet when he sees one.[34]

I want to look at one more Victorian treatment of women and clothing, one that suggests a compelling reason why the self-contained world of fashion might be censured so rigorously. Elizabeth Gaskell's novel *North and South* opens with one of the few positive scenes of female self-admiration in the nineteenth-century canon. Its heroine, Margaret Hale, models cashmere shawls before a mirror, taking an obviously sensuous pleasure in the process. Regarding her beautiful reflection with "a quiet pleased smile on her lips," Margaret basks in the delights of her costume: "their spicy eastern smell . . . their soft feel and their brilliant colours."[35] When Henry Lennox, her soon-to-be-suitor, enters the room, she displays "not a tinge of shyness or self-consciousness," not having yet learned to be embarrassed by her sartorial appreciation (though her older aunts are "half-ashamed of their feminine interest in dress") or to connect it with sexual availability (10, 9). Margaret's pleasure in these scenes is at once innocent and sensual, self-contained and completely lacking in the sexual predation that the coquette is supposed to practice. Lennox is not the real viewer for whom she rehearses her self-presentation; she does not adorn herself to attract men. The scene is a prelapsarian idyll consisting of a woman, her reflection, and her clothes.[36] With their autoerotic appeal, cashmere shawls seems to signify Margaret's self-contained indifference to male admiration: the first time she meets Thornton, whom she weds after a prolonged, painful relationship, she wears her own cashmere shawl "as an empress wears her drapery" (62), with "no awkwardness" (61), and greets Thornton with "a simple, straight, unabashed look" (62). Thornton is, in contrast, "surprised and discomfited" by her appearance (61). In both scenes, Gaskell contrasts Margaret's style, which is beautiful but does not aim at seduction, with male desire, marking the gap between them.

The rest of the novel destroys Margaret's self-containment, replacing it with the much more complicated and often traumatic experience of heterosexuality. In a series of paradigmatic moments, Margaret's image is repeatedly wrested from her own vision and placed in the sightline of sexualizing gazes, which rewrite her body as an erotic object and fill her with the shame she so conspicuously lacked before the mirror. Henry's proposal, which leaves her "guilty and ashamed of having grown so much into a woman to be thought of in marriage," prepares the way for more brutal experiences (32–33). The famous strike scene, in which Margaret uses her body to shield the mill owner Thornton from striking workers, opens her publicly to unwelcome sexual meanings, as others assume that her behavior has betrayed her love—including Thornton, who quickly declares his own feelings.[37] In a second scene, a clandestine walk with her fugitive brother leads once again to the public assumption that Margaret is tainted with desire. While both of these assumptions are false in their details, Margaret cannot erase their more general effects of producing her as a sexual body available to men and making her ashamed of her beauty.[38]

The aftermath of the strike scene clarifies the self-alienation that forms the necessary precondition to Margaret's heterosexuality. When she thinks of Thornton's proposal, she feels the "cold slime" of sexual innuendo and has a dreamlike vision of the shame that attends her development:

The deep impression made by that interview [in which she is accused of loving Thornton], was like that of a horror in a dream, that will not leave the room although we waken up, and rub our eyes, and force a stiff, rigid smile upon our lips. It is there—there, cowering and gibbering, with fixed ghastly eyes, in some corner of the chamber, listening to hear whether we dare breathe of its presence to anyone. (198)

The delectable image of her own body draped in luxurious shawls has given way to horror, as Thornton's desire, invading her psychic space, produces a new female sexuality that is alien, uncanny, demonic. Margaret must learn to relinquish her untroubled, self-contained pleasure for her role as the object of male admiration; unable to control her effect on others, she is nevertheless ashamed of beauty. Perhaps reflecting this discomfort, Margaret has no relationship to her clothing by the end of the novel. Before the dinner party that reunites Margaret with Thornton, Margaret's maid lays out her dress and her cousin chooses her flowers while Margaret is out, without her participation. When Margaret agrees to marry Thornton, her face is "glowing with a beautiful shame," the mark of the properly heterosexual woman (436). Although this is clearly her happy ending, the novel registers an uncompromising recognition of what she sacrifices in this forced march toward femininity, and quite surprisingly locates her sunniest erotic moment in communion with clothing and her own image. As in the cautionary tale about the extravagant narcissist, heterosexuality competes with the rewards of fashion, but *North and South* articulates the stakes of the contest: female agency and pleasure. Margaret must accept a painful self-alienation as the price of "normal" development.

What is implicit in the treatments of fashion that I have discussed and comes closest to explicit expression in *North and South* is that attacks on coquetry are a kind of cover story that conceals less familiar fears about gender roles and heterosexuality, and above all about female authority, autonomy, and eroticism. In "Good Looks," one of its essays on fashion, *Cornhill Magazine* reassures readers that "woman commits no idolatry herself: she does not worship her own loveliness—she only gives opportunity for others to do so," but its own repeated colonializing of fashion under the rubric of historical knowledge signals a certain unease about how completely the heterosexual imperative controlled women's self-adornment.[39] A reservoir of skill and knowledge might lurk beneath this unassuming loveliness, granting women an unacknowledged authority over aesthetic practices and social relations. And of course in dismissing the question of women's "idolatry," *Cornhill Magazine* also raises it, with a word choice that hints at not only seductiveness but also the more dangerous crime of self-worship. Behind the code word "vanity," which points our attention at the familiar dyad of the manipulative beauty and her male victim, lie other, even more subversive pairings: the woman and her milliner, the woman and her clothing, the woman and her own image. Ironically, the come-hither glance is the least of the coquette's sins. It is her inward gaze, dazzled by her own finery, that scandalizes fashion moralists.

Notes

1. We can see a modem version of the fashion double bind in the psychiatric diagnosis of "female dressing disorder," understood as the individual pathology of teenage girls who are obsessed with their appearance and not as the result of a cultural mandate. See Efrat Tseëlon, *The Masque of Femininity: The Presentation of Women in Everyday Life* (London: Sage, 1995), 17.

2. Margaret Oliphant, *Dress* (Philadelphia: Porter and Coates, 1879), 81; Alexander Walker, *Woman Physiologically Considered as to Mind, Morals, Marriage, Matrimonial Slavery, Infidelity, and Divorce* (London: Simkin, Marshall and Co., 1840), xi; Eliza Haweis, *The Art of Beauty and the Art of Dress* (Reprint, New York and London: Garland, 1978), 9.

3. Walker, 50. Subsequent quotations will be cited parenthetically in the text. For a discussion of the tenuous Victorian distinction between "honest dress" and "finery," the latter was linked pervasively to immorality and the fallen woman; see Mariana Valverde, "The Love of Finery: Fashion and the Fallen Woman in Nineteenth-Century Social Discourse," *Victorian Studies* 32, no. 2 (1989): 168–88.

4. Claire Walsh, "The Newness of the Department Store: A View from the Eighteenth Century," in *Cathedrals of Consumption: The European Department Store, 1850–1939,* ed. Geoffrey Crossick and Serge Jaumain (Aldershot, England: Ashgate, 1999), 46.

5. This phrase is borrowed from Erika Diane Rappaport, *Shopping for Pleasure: Women and the Making of London's West End* (Princeton: Princeton University Press, 2000).

6. Laurel Brake and Julie F. Codell, eds. *Encounters in the Victorian Press: Editors, Authors, Readers* (Hampshire, England: Palgrave Macmillan, 2005), 2. As Margaret Beetham points out in *A Magazine of Her Own? Domesticity and Desire in the Woman's Magazine, 1800–1914* (London: Routledge, 1996), the *Waterloo Directory* includes over 29,000 titles of periodicals published between 1824 and 1900. For accounts of the technological changes that made this explosion of journals possible, see Richard D. Altick, *The English Common Reader: A Social History of the Mass Reading Public, 1800–1900* (Columbus: Ohio State University Press, 1998) and Patricia Anderson, *The Printer Image and the Transformation of Popular Culture, 1790–1860* (Oxford: Oxford University Press, 1991).

7. Beetham, *A Magazine of Her Own*, 40. Beetham provides an extensive examination of women's magazines in the nineteenth and early twentieth centuries, including fashion magazines. She sees the 1830s and 1840s as a foundational moment in the development of high-end, fashion-focused periodicals.

8. Margaret Oliphant observes, "The fashion' in man's apparel, though it goes on shifting and changing as well as the other, has so veiled and sheltered itself under the greater pretensions of the feminine toilette, that no one takes any notice of it." Oliphant, *Dress*, 64–65. For an extended scholarly analysis of the ways in which fashionable men's clothing continued to be promoted, see Brent Shannon, *The Cut of His Coat: Men, Dress, and Consumer Culture in Britain, 1860–1914* (Athens: Ohio University Press, 2006).

9. Alexander Walker, *Beauty in Woman Analysed and Classified with a Critical View of the Hypotheses of the Most Eminent Writers, Painters, and Sculptors* (London: Simkin, Marshall, and Co., 1892). I treat Walker's arguments about the coquette's sexual threat and his self-presentation as an expert in a more extended discussion of his work in my *Unauthorized Pleasures: Accounts of Victorian Erotic Experience* (Ithaca, NY: Cornell University Press, 2003), 60–72.

10. "Colours for Female Dress." *Ladies' Pocket Magazine* 13 (1830): 64.

11. For a complex and extended discussion of theories of the everyday, see Laurie Langbauer, *Novels of Everyday Life: The Series in English Fiction, 1850–1930* (Ithaca, NY: Cornell University Press, 1999), especially pages 19–23, where she examines and contests Lefebvre's influential assertion that women have an especially intimate and uncritical relationship to the everyday.

12. Haweis, *The Art of Beauty and the Art of Dress*, 14.

13. See, for instance, Anne Hollander's *Seeing Through Clothes* (New York: Viking, 1978), where she asserts that "dress is a form of visual art" (311) and analyzes self-adornment as a form of portraiture (392). See also Valerie Steele, *Fashion and Eroticism: Ideals of Feminine Beauty from the Victorian Era to the Jazz Age* (Oxford: Oxford University Press, 1985).

14. Hollander, in *Seeing Through Clothes*, notes the influence of canonical portraits and paintings on popular fashion illustrations (315–16).

15. Indeed, in *Dress*, Margaret Oliphant complained that fashion might have veered a bit too close to art in its temporary adaptation of the Greek *chyton*; one might just as well recommend togas for men, she observes dryly (67–68).

16. Charles Dickens, *Bleak House* (Harmondsworth: Penguin, 1998), 138. For discussions of the fashion plate and women's magazines, see Kay Boardman, "'A Material Girl in a Material World': The Fashionable Female Body in Victorian Women's Magazines," *Journal of Victorian Culture* 3 (1998): 93–110 (especially 98–99); and Beetham, *A Magazine of Her Own?*, who notes the circulation of Lady Dedlock's image in this context (especially 36–41).

17. Hollander, *Seeing Through Clothes*, 316. Hollander asserts that the appropriation worked both ways, because paintings of historical subjects sometimes adopted the clothing conventions of their own period.

18. "Beautiful For Ever," *Dublin University Magazine* 81 (March 1873): 301–11. This title may have been a direct appropriation, since it was also the name of the beauty salon owned by the infamous Rachel Leverson, who combined selling cosmetics and extortion in an extremely lucrative business until she was convicted of fraud in 1868.

19. "Aesthetics of Dress," *Blackwood's* 57, February 1945, 243.

20. Many scholars have traced the rise of scientific medicine in the nineteenth century, as surgeons, who underwent formal scientific training, competed for the cultural capital that was formerly vested in gentleman physicians, whose classical education and concentration on internal ailments signified their higher social status. For a summary, see Rosenman, *Unauthorized Pleasures*, 27–30.

21. For an account of the correspondence about tight lacing in *The English-woman's Domestic Magazine*, see Beetham, *A Magazine of Her Own?*, 81–88.

22. "Fashion," *Chambers's Journal of Popular Literature, Science, and Art*, 4th Series, 19 (13 May, 1882): 297.

23. George Henry Lewes, "Aids to Beauty, Real and Artificial," *Cornhill Magazine* 7, March 1863, 392.

24. J. Milner Fothergill, MD, "Fashions and Physiology," *Good Words* 23 (February 1882): 136.

25. The well-known flâneur and diarist Arthur Munby complained repeatedly about pert shopgirls. See Derek Hudson, *Munby. Man of Two Worlds: The Life and Diaries of Arthur J. Munby, 1828–1910* (New York: Gambit, 1972), 60–61. For a detailed account of the shopgirl's significance as a symbol of modernity and consumer culture at the end of the century, see Lisa Shapiro Sanders, *Consuming Fantasies: Labor, Leisure, and the London Shopgirl, 1880–1920* (Columbus: The Ohio State University Press, 2006).

26. "Shops, Shopkeepers, Shopmen, and Shop Morality," *Edinburgh Journal* 14 (1850), 162.

27. Quoted in C. Willis Cunnington and Phyllis Cunnington, *Handbook of English Costume in the Nineteenth Century* (London: Faber and Faber, 1959), 14.

28. "Dress in Paris," *All the Year Round* 9 (February 28, 1863), 9. The article also notes the existence of an Englishman who has perfected the design and fitting of stays but who remains "in other respects a perfect gentleman" (9).

29. Cunnington and Cunnington, *Handbook of English Costume*, 14.

30. Margaret Beetham's analysis in *A Magazine of Her Own?* of the controversy over corsets in the *Englishwoman's Domestic Magazine* reveals tension between heterosexuality and autoerotic desire. While several correspondents condemn women for undergoing the dangerous torture of tight lacing and others fear that male readers may read the magazine as a kind of pornography, at least one correspondent (anonymous, so perhaps male) writes of the corporeal pleasures of tight lacing. Beetham argues that this subject, and women's magazines in general, repeatedly register the tension between "a sexuality of 'sensation'" and "a sexuality of 'the gaze'" (87).

31. "Dress in Paris," 9.

32. George Eliot, *Daniel Deronda* (Harmondsworth: Penguin, 1967), 47.

33. Jean Baudrillard, *Seduction*, trans. Brian Singer (New York: St. Martin's Press, 1990), 86.

34. Hollander, *Seeing Through Clothes*, 311.

35. Elizabeth Gaskell, *North and South* (Oxford: Oxford University Press, 1982), 9. Although Suzanne Daly asserts that Margaret's shawl is "largely stripped" of its link to the exotic east, this description evokes the sensual, Orientalist associations that Daly details in her essay, "Kashmir Shawls in mid-Victorian Novels," *Victorian Literature and Culture* 30 (2002): 249. Daly's reading of the shawl in

North and South illuminates its role in the context of English manufacturing and industrialism (249–51).

36. In this context, it may not be too fanciful to allude to *Sex and the City*, with its emphasis on the ecstasy of shopping, dressing, and homosocial bonding, and its reluctance, in its television version, to provide the happy heterosexual ending of marriage for Carrie, its central character. As for the movie, in spite of its resolution in Carrie's marriage, critics blasted the superficial pleasures of its characters. In *Newsweek*, Ramin Setoodeh calls this reaction "Sexism in the City," noting cogently, "What's surprising is the length guys have gone to push Carrie off her Manolos." Ramin Setoodeh, "Sexism and *Sex and the City*," *Newsweek*, June 16, 2008, 46.

37. Although a number of critics agree, I can see no evidence for this in the text. See Rosemarie Bodenheimer, *The Politics of Story in Victorian Social Fiction* (Ithaca, NY: Cornell University Press, 1988), 66; Patsy Stoneman, *Elizabeth Gaskell* (Bloomington: Indiana University Press, 1987), 129; Barbara Leah Harman, "In Promiscuous Company: Female Public Appearance in Elizabeth Gaskell's *North and South*," *Victorian Studies* 31, no. 3 (Spring 1988), 369; Deborah Nord, *Walking the Victorian Streets: Women, Representation, and the City* (Ithaca, NY: Cornell University Press, 1995), 174.

38. See also Nord, *Walking the Victorian Streets*. She notes that *North and South* suggests "how powerful, how unavoidable, was the sexualization of woman's entry into [public urban] space" (176).

39. "Good Looks," *Cornhill Magazine* 14, September 1866, 339.

Kara Tennant

❦ 5

THE DISCERNING EYE

Viewing the Mid-Victorian "Modern" Woman

The Modern Spectator

In the mid 1870s, the French painter Jean Béraud produced a work in oils entitled *Parisienne un jour de pluie, place de la Concorde*.[1] The painting depicts a young woman, who appears to have paused momentarily in the street. With her left hand she holds a black umbrella over her shoulder and with her right, she lifts her skirts delicately off the wet ground. From underneath her red hat, which matches her red stockings and the red trim on her sleeve, she looks out, boldly meeting the gaze of the viewer. Her expression is difficult to read; it is not clear whether she invites or combats our inquisitive glance, whether our presence is welcomed or intrusive. Her clothing, too, is ambiguous. She wears a gray-and-white dress, discreetly flounced, yet also hinting at richness and even coquetry. While the painting exquisitely renders the color and texture of contemporary dress, we cannot determine whether her costume indicates a lady who is modishly up-to-date with the fashions, or if her outfit may suggest a less reputable occupation. Although we see a gentleman in the background who, like the central figure, stops and stares, he is not sufficiently close for us to determine whether he meets our gaze or if he, like us, focuses upon the young woman. The more we look at the painting, the more it beguiles us, and the more it evades a single, stable reading.

The multiple possibilities for interpretation suggested by Béraud's painting are connected with more fundamental issues about viewing and display, which, as I will explore in this chapter, become inextricably linked with mid-Victorian understandings of clothing, femininity, and the cultural condition that became known as "modernity." These issues may lead us to consider that, while the visual could clarify and elucidate, it could also obfuscate and deny any straightforward "truth" or meaning. In *The*

Victorians and the Visual Imagination, Kate Flint addresses these matters as she contemplates the problematic centrality of the visual to Victorian culture as a whole. She suggests that "[t]he Victorians were fascinated with the act of seeing, with the question of the reliability—or otherwise—of the human eye, and with the problems of interpreting what they saw."[2] Flint argues that Victorian visual practices were concerned with "bringing things to the surface . . . making things available to the eye and hence ready for interpretation."[3] But, as she shows, the very act of interpretation is not in itself straightforward, as visual signifiers could also be misleading. Indeed, in *Techniques of the Observer*, Jonathan Crary identifies the mid-to-late nineteenth century as a period during which the notion of objective vision gave way to a sense that perception could be subjective and partial. He argues that "any single medium or form of visual representation no longer has a significant autonomous identity" and that neither image nor "observer" could be separated from their "overloaded and plural sensory environment."[4]

What Crary describes is more than just a development in nineteenth-century viewing practices, and represents part of a much wider cultural phenomenon. He asserts that, during this period, the observer becomes part of a "process of modernization," during which he or she is subject "to a constellation of new events, forces, and institutions that together are loosely and perhaps tautologically definable as 'modernity.'"[5] The very notion of the modern is closely associated with Charles Baudelaire's 1863 essay "The Painter of Modern Life." Baudelaire identifies the idea of modernity in the work of Constantin Guys or "Monsieur G.," an artist who, like Béraud, views and sketches everyday scenes of nineteenth-century Paris and, in doing so, captures "universal life."[6] Part of Monsieur G.'s artistry, Baudelaire suggests, lies in the subtle discernment of sartorial changes, and upon his intimate familiarity with the visual vocabulary of female clothing:

[I]f a fashion or the cut of a garment has been slightly modified, if bows and curls have been supplanted by cockades, if *bavolets* have been enlarged and chignons have dropped a fraction towards the nape of the neck, if waists have been raised and skirts have become fuller, be very sure that his eagle eye will already have spotted it from however great a distance.[7]

Through his subtle discernment of sartorial changes, Monsieur G. captures the manifestation of contemporary fashion within urban life in a witty, dynamic manner. In celebrating this technique, Baudelaire's essay suggests that fashion demarcates the modern and is perpetuated by it. For

Baudelaire, clothing punctuates, defines, and is inseparable from the "universal life" of modernity.

Around this time, however, another, very different, discourse addressing clothing and the modern—or, indeed, modern clothing—emerged, and it is upon this that I will focus throughout this chapter. For the term "modernity" also started to appear in popular fiction, journalism, and cultural commentaries of the 1860s, and—unlike Baudelaire's rhetoric, which evoked *la modernité* with a sense of wonder and reverence—was often used as a means of "branding" or condemning less traditional elements of fashionable culture. This interpretation of the modern performs a radically different function to that conceived by Baudelaire, and was frequently used to foreground ideological issues associated with social class, femininity, and sexuality, reading clothing and fashionable comportment as visual signifiers of the declining moral and aesthetic impact of contemporary women's fashion standards. For this reason, I draw upon a broad range of illustrated and visual texts, discussing widely read journalistic material such as Mrs. Eliza Lynn Linton's notorious "Girl of the Period" articles, which proposed an alarming new understanding of modern female fashion and behaviors, alongside less familiar publications such as the *Girl of the Period Almanack* and the *Girl of the Period Miscellany*, which satirized "modern" womanhood while simultaneously exposing its subversions and complexities.

Through an examination of contemporary novels, journalism, and periodicals, I will also examine the dynamics of display, observation, and interpretation, which are of central importance to the mid-century modern. Indeed, the mid-Victorian period is well known for its social mechanisms designed for the viewing and evaluation of female clothing and comportment. Yet, within this framework it would seem that there was not always an acknowledged position for the female spectator. This issue is explored in the anonymous 1860 novel *Grandmother's Money*, which addresses the position of the female viewer of contemporary women's fashion.[8] This novel asserts the significance of the informed female viewer, instructing the reader in how to interpret sartorial cues, but simultaneously undermining the widely held notion that to see was also to discern. With this in mind, I will finally turn to Mrs. Ellen Wood's 1861 "sensation" novel *East Lynne*, which, alongside Mrs. Linton's series of articles, also foregrounds the ambiguities of viewing associated with "modern" womanhood. What emerges, I suggest, is a sense of disjunction between the visual and the moral, which cannot be mediated through traditional understandings of "old" and "new" femininity.

Clothing and Readability

During the nineteenth century, the notion that clothing should be clearly readable was widely accepted. An anonymous American guidebook entitled *A Manual of Politeness*, published in 1837, suggests that a lady's clothing may be understood as "a very intelligible index of the wearer's well-regulated mind."[9] Indeed, the author observes that they "never yet met with a woman whose general style of dress was chaste, elegant, and appropriate, that [they] did not find, on further acquaintance, to be, in disposition and mind, an object to admire and love."[10] The notion of dress as a readily readable "index" recurs in Mrs. Matilda Pullan's 1855 *Maternal Counsels to a Daughter*, in which she describes the "attire" as "so unfailing" and "so accurate" as an "index of the mind" that she claims that "we need little more than a single glance at a woman to be able to learn all the most salient points in her character."[11] We see a similar ideology at work twelve years later, in 1867, when the *Saturday Review* journalist Mrs. Linton claimed that dress ought to be "individual and symbolic, so as to indicate clearly the position and character which we desire to obtain and hold."[12] Yet, during the 1860s, new modes of fashionable costume and behavior were emerging, which challenged the notion that clothing could be read as a series of "codes" that unproblematically corresponded with different social classes or moral ideologies.

The 1860s have been criticized, as Doris Langley Moore points out, for their "fast and vulgar manners."[13] Likewise, Valerie Steele describes contemporary dress as "garish," arguing that the period's "complex construction, bright colors, and elaboration were intended to produce a rich and opulent yet feminine and coquettish effect."[14] In August 1860, *Punch* magazine published a gleefully satirical verse entitled "Fast Young Ladies,"[15] which caricatured new trends in female behavior. The poem describes a "flashy set," identifiable by the feathers in their hats, their "hitched up" skirts, flame-colored petticoats, and "high-heeled boots," sartorial features that serve to emphasize their brash, brazen demeanor. The misogyny typified by *Punch* was also echoed in publications aimed specifically at women. In November 1862, the "Society" column of the *Ladies' Newspaper* printed a series of letters from both male and female readers addressing the "fast" behavior of young men and women, which also construct a reciprocal relationship between modern clothing and lowering standards of female comportment.

On November 22, 1862, a letter was published entitled "Fast People and Domestic Habits" from a correspondent named "Minnie," who concurs with a previous reader that "the young men and women of the pres-

ent time are a great deal too fast in their habits and manners."[16] "Minnie"
interprets this as both a class and a gender issue, observing that she
"should like to see some of the lower middle classes, tradesmen's wives
and daughters a little more attentive to domestic duties, instead of flying
about, dressed out in such a ridiculous manner as they do." The "natural
consequence" of this, the writer implies, is ultimately the denigration of
domestic life, namely "family disputes and discomfort, and very often
ruin to the children." In this way, modern dress is not only visually disturbing, but is connected with the decline of moral values and the dete-
rioration of the home.

The Girl of the Period

As "Minnie's" letter suggests, the sense of outrage and ridicule frequently
associated with "modern" dress seems indicative of a radical redefinition
of fashionable femininity. Mrs. Linton's infamous "The Girl of the Period" article appeared in the *Saturday Review* on March 14, 1868, and
made a vitriolic attack on both female dress and fashionable comportment, linking these directly with a sense of the contemporary and the
"modern." The article introduced the character of the Girl of the Period
herself, whose brightly colored, impractical wardrobe spoke clearly of
her desire to flirt with men and to push the boundaries of "respectable"
conduct. In a much quoted passage from this article, we are told that

[t]he girl of the period is a creature who dyes her hair and paints her face, as
the first articles of her personal religion; whose sole idea of life is plenty of fun
and luxury; and whose dress is the object of such thought and intellect as she
possesses.[17]

Often cited as an example of Victorian "antimodern" rhetoric, Mrs. Linton characterizes this new feminine type as a "loud and rampant modernization," sporting "false red hair and painted skin," physical characteristics that reflect the dubious morals of the demimondaine that she
supposedly imitated (340).

The article establishes a conflict between "old" and "new" modes of
femininity. Mrs. Linton creates a figurative gulf between the Girl of the
Period and the "fair young English girl of the past," who, she writes, represents "the ideal of womanhood [. . .] of home birth, and breeding" and
who is "content to be what God and nature had made [her]."[18] In contrast, the Girl of the Period becomes a visual personification of the modern in all its brashness, extravagance, and indecency, which, Mrs. Linton
claims in another article, "makes the present state of things so deplorable."[19]

In this piece, published on May 9, 1868, she constructs a reciprocal dependence between personal adornment and the self-interest of modern womanhood, arguing that "the ideal woman of truth and modesty and simple love and homely living has somehow faded away under the paint and tinsel of this modern reality."[20]

Although Mrs. Linton presents the Girl of the Period as a contemporary, urgent problem, we see a similar conception of femininity presented some years earlier, in Wilkie Collins's 1852 novel, *Basil*. In this novel, the eponymous narrator's sister, Clara, seems to function as a prototype for Mrs. Linton's "old English ideal": she is described as "the kind, gentle, happy young English girl, who could enter into everybody's interests, and be grateful for everybody's love," who, "in her own quiet, natural manner" was "always the presiding spirit of general comfort and general friendship."[21] Significantly, Clara's naturalness and "simplicity" are favorably juxtaposed with another kind of Englishwoman; the very type, in fact, of whom Mrs. Linton writes some sixteen years later. Indeed, Basil is explicitly concerned that ladies will lose their traditionally "feminine" qualities, writing that

[w]e live in an age when too many women appear to be ambitious of morally unsexing themselves before society, by aping the language and the manners of men [. . .] Women of this exclusively modern order, like to use slang expressions in their conversation; assume a bastard-masculine abruptness in their manners, a bastard-masculine license in their opinions [. . .] [n]othing impresses, agitates, amuses, or delights them in a hearty, natural, womanly way. Sympathy looks ironical, if they ever show it: love seems to be an affair of calculation, or mockery, or contemptuous sufferance, if they ever feel it.[22]

While Collins's narrator is anxious to preserve a more traditional model of femininity, he seems significantly less concerned than Mrs. Linton with "modern" clothing. Rather, Collins's novel emphasizes a worryingly unfeminine trend in female comportment, which the narrator associates with a lack of "genuine" feeling. In Basil's terms, "natural, womanly" values are replaced with a false or superficial emotional engagement, which is, curiously, aligned with masculinity.

The masculine elements of the "modern" woman were widely satirized in a spin-off series of magazines that was published by the anonymous editor "Miss Echo" of London, in response to Mrs. Linton's "Girl of the Period" series. A magazine entitled the *Girl of the Period Almanack* appeared in 1869, and was followed by the *Girl of the Period Miscellany* in the same year, which ran for nine issues. A second (and final) *Almanack* was published in 1870. The 1869 *Almanack* features a cartoon for every month of the year, accompanied by an explanatory text in the form of a letter from a number of recurring characters including "Lilly White," "Polly Glott," and "Flora Gardens." The illustrations have humorous and provocative titles such as "The Pallas Billiard Club" (February), "The Alcyone Angling Club" (April) and "The Syren Flirting Club" (December). Each depicts a group of ladies wearing recognizably "fast" dress, who are shown undertaking a variety of traditionally male activities. Or, in Hilary Fraser, Stephanie Green, and Judith Johnston's terms, we see "a variety of smoking, drinking, immodestly attired young hoydens engaged in a range of athletic, fast, and unfeminine pursuits."[23]

It is fascinating that, in these illustrations, excessively ornamented and elaborate feminine clothing is aligned with activities that are both "fast" and explicitly masculine. The women's dress is juxtaposed with their exaggeratedly "masculine" postures as they lounge on benches, make bets on horses, and stand, smoking cigarettes and with their hands on their hips. In the illustration entitled "The Pallas Billiard Club," one "girl" waits, holding her billiard cue upright, while another plays her shot (figure 5.1). This woman leans over the table, her body precisely poised and her eyes downturned in serious concentration. Describing this scene, the character "Lilly White" writes:

You can easily understand that, as a posture game, we find billiards invaluable. Every variety of attitude, every grace, every calisthenic perfection may be indulged in whilst leaning over the table. Anon the captivating bend of the long reach forces me into the lovely pose of the flying nymph, and presently that difficult stroke with the cue behind my back—the despair of the gawky and fat—forces me into the die-away lassitude of the swooning Bacchante. My success has been immense![24]

Somewhat paradoxically, this lady's masculine comportment, along with her participation in the traditionally male pursuit of billiards, only serves to emphasize her lithe female physicality and erotic appeal. While she describes herself in traditionally feminine terms as "lovely" and "captivating," this is combined with a self-awareness and a sense of sexual daring that is both reinforced and undermined by the series of pseudo-classical "pose[s]" that she adopts as she undertakes the game.

This contradiction between masculinity and femininity is visually dramatized in the illustration. The stance of the woman on the left affords not only a full view of the front of her jacket and blouse, but also of the detail on the back of her outfit.[25] She wears a ruched skirt looped up over a petticoat trimmed with a deep ruffle, while her single-breasted jacket opens to reveal a spotted blouse with an upturned collar, lending

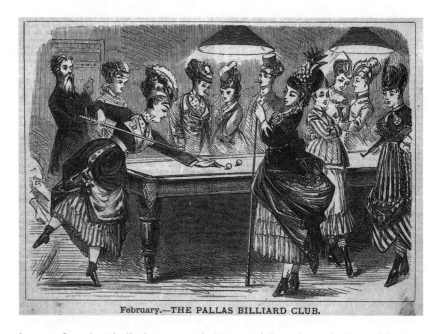

February.—THE PALLAS BILLIARD CLUB.

her outfit a decidedly humorously "mannish" quality, which starkly juxtaposes with the frills and ruffles with which her skirts are embellished. In addition, the absurdity of the ladies' behavior is reinforced through small sartorial details, as their outfits are complemented by themed accessories that wryly undermine the ladies' serious concentration on their activities. The billiard-playing lady's jacket is drawn together with a horseshoe-shaped belt, while the ladies in March's illustration, "The Circe Betting Club," wear horseshoe earrings and clothing adorned with a similar motif. In the June cartoon, "The Hero Rowing Club," one woman wears a flat headpiece in the shape of a target, impaled with decorative arrows, while a cigarette-smoking, belligerent-looking lady has decorated her coiffure with an ornamental anchor that hangs from the back of her chignon. Although the anchor, arrow, and horseshoe were popular symbols in jewelry during the period, in these cartoons, the illustrator lends them a buoyant, jaunty character that serves to emphasize the ladies' humorously errant behavior.[26]

Although the women wear elaborate dress, their clothing does not inhibit them from ice-skating, playing billiards, fishing in a boat, or jostling one another on the football pitch. In "The Thetis Yachting Club," Georgie Shelley takes pride both in her appearance and her sailing ability. She boasts that she and her companion, Miss Willie Luxmoore, look "uncommonly well" in their "smart pea-jackets with gilt buttons," and that they also are "of great use on board," being "always ready to bear a hand, to belay, to avast, to go up aloft, to ready-about, or anything [they] are called upon to do." The letter concludes with a contemptuous dismissal of "those fresh-water girls who do nothing but sport the Club buttons and eat the Club's preserved provisions on dry land."[27] Indeed, Georgie perceives the "Club buttons" as more than a mere accoutrement, implying that those who adopt the nautical uniform should also be willing to adopt the vigorous, implicitly masculine lifestyle that it denotes. Yet the pseudo-masculine tone of the narrative, with its overuse of sailing terminology, not only implicitly ridicules the Girl of the Period's nautical pretensions but also serves to remind the reader of a more traditional model of femininity against which she can be offset and evaluated.[28]

The final epistle for 1869, "The Syren Flirting Club," explicitly presents a condemnatory perspective on the Girl of the Period. Rather than being authored by one of the young women, the letter is attributed to an outside observer, "Mrs. Fanny Roseneath," an older lady who hosts "nine unpleasant guests" over the Christmas season. She describes how "these gaudy dolls infest [her] home," offending "[e]steemed friends" with their rowdy talk, and creating "merriment" with their "fashionable toilettes."[29] She claims that

[r]eprehensible in the extreme is their style of dress, when in full array, so bold and undisguised that my dear husband was modestly moved. The hair is so managed with stuffings and puffings that it towers and juts to the size of a lard bladder; the full shoulders spread over a tight-laced bodice, so small in proportion, it is but as a bouquet holder, and thus girdled, not clothed, they sit on show, encouraging, by their bold glances, the advances of men.

Unlike her husband, who is only "modestly moved," Mrs. Roseneath makes connections between "fast" clothing and flirtatious behavior, reading dress as a visual symptom of her guests' dubious morality. By this logic, both modish clothing and the attempt to attract the opposite sex are, somewhat paradoxically, portrayed as unfeminine, ridiculous, and socially inappropriate. But, as if oblivious of the effect she has upon the male and female observer, the Girl of the Period perceives herself as progressive rather than defiant; Lilly White concludes, "we are rather fast, but certainly not vulgar."[30]

In the *Girl of the Period Miscellany*, clothing is equally conspicuous and overbearing. Its very first article, which describes a meeting "in the Editorial Sanctum," quickly moves into a discussion of costume, making an implicit condemnation of the character of "Miss Flora Gardens." This lady appears "dressed in a corded silk of emerald green, ruched to death; corsage veiled à la provoquante, and emerald-green silk boots, perched on emerald-green heels as tall as dice-boxes." She looks, we are told, "green and fresh as spring grass after a shower."[31] In another article, provocatively entitled "What is the Girl of the Period For?" this feminine type is depicted as a vigorous-looking young woman wearing a striped dress that is embellished with a horseshoe design and arranged so as to expose her frilled petticoat and buttoned boots. Suspended from her dress is a long, poker-like umbrella, while a round hat, adorned with a veil and a stuffed, long-tailed bird, awkwardly rests against her large chignon. Carrying a sizeable beribboned fur muff, she walks purposefully forward, scrutinizing the scene ahead through *pince-nez*.[32] This daunting visual image, with its curious, humorous blend of strident masculinity and female fashionability, draws attention to the inherent contradictions embodied by this conception of "modern" womanhood.

Although the article initially dismisses the Girl of the Period as "the masculine Giggle of the Hour," we may also infer hidden complications. For "if we look closely," as the writer suggests, we may discover that "she is not such a mere weed as she has been made out to be."[33] In this way, as Fraser et al have suggested, the *Miscellany* insidiously exposes the "limitations" of Mrs. Linton's original character. They argue that the Girl of the Period, rather than having a single, coherent identity, is in fact a "multiform being" who engages in activities as diverse as croquet, sailing, hunting, ballet, millinery, serving refreshments, and factory work.[34] Indeed, the first issue of the *Miscellany* divides the Girl of the Period into smaller, increasingly specific subsets according to occupation, such as "The Ballet Girl," "The Refreshment-Bar Girl," and "The Sewing-Machine Girl."[35] These cartoons, unlike those featured in the *Almanack*, do not draw upon a coherent illustrative style, implicitly challenging the notion that the Girl of the Period can be interpreted as one recognizable "type."

Unlike the *Almanack*, in which the illustrations are bold and readily readable, the *Miscellany* presents interesting disjunctions between image and text. The illustration of "The Sewing-Machine Girl," for example, portrays an attractive, clean-looking young woman who is smartly but not showily dressed, and situated within a seemingly domestic setting that thus blurs the boundaries between home and workplace. In this sense, illustration and verse complement each another to construct an impression of industriousness and contentment; not only does she "sing and stitch with a merry sound," but that she is "[h]appy and gay as a summer's queen." Yet, the verse also informs the reader that this respectably dressed, chaste-looking lady also finds time "[t]o prattle, smile and flirt"—behavior that is not even hinted at in the picture. The Sewing-Machine Girl's meaningless flirtation reminds us of the unreliability of the visual image and specifically of the image of the demure woman. In this way, the piece also functions as a reminder that, within many different contexts, women were subject to continual scrutiny and evaluation for the way in which they presented themselves.

Observing Fashion

The literature of the mid-nineteenth century regularly articulates the importance of "seeing and being seen." In the summer of 1862, the periodical *London Society* published an illustrated two-part series entitled "Fashionable Promenades," which featured an article entitled "Brighton—In and Out of Season" in its July issue, and a poem, "In Kensington Gardens," the following month, in August. The latter evokes a lighthearted fashionable scene as ladies and gentlemen promenade through the gardens in order "to laugh and to listen, to see and be seen"—a familiar concept for the fashion-conscious reader.[36] The verse closely links the display and viewing of clothing with the acts of flirtation and courtship; the ladies, we are told, not only wish to display "their silks and their laces," but also hope to "inveigle the men in the park from their studies and stools." In the penultimate stanza, the cheerful band music provides a backdrop for a more meaningful interplay of "glances" and "answering looks" that, we infer, may lead to a declaration of love. In his 1862 novel *Orley Farm*, Anthony Trollope confirms this poem's depiction of the dynamics of fashionable viewing practices. The novel's narrator claims that each and every social event is an occasion for the viewing of female beauty, reflecting that, even on a rural hunting excursion, "the object is pretty much the same here as in the ballroom. 'Spectatum veniunt; veniunt spectentuer ut ipsæ,' as it is proper, natural, and desirable that they should do."[37]

Even the poor and provincial Barbara Bloyce, the "paid companion" in the anonymous 1860 novel *Grandmother's Money*, recognizes the social significance of such fashionable display.[38] The novel follows Barbara as she leaves her Jersey home to work for the wealthy and cantankerous Mrs. Tresdaile. While the action is largely based in London, a significant section of the first volume takes place at the popular seaside resort of Hastings, where Barbara's elderly employer has been ordered to go as a rest cure. On walking the pier for the first time, accompanied by Mrs. Tresdaile and her niece, Alice, Barbara wryly observes that

[t]he Fashionables or the Unfashionables were riding by in their broughams, or cantering gaily past on horseback, or going out for a sail, or making for the beach and the bathing machines. It was a bright sunny morning; Hastings

seemed full of life and activity, and Alice thought she should like to live there, "oh! for ever and ever!"[39]

Though Barbara "would have preferred hill, dale and corn-field" to the lively scene before her, she is conscious of the importance that the younger woman places on participating in fashionable seaside culture, easily discerning Alice's delight at "the Parade, the music and the gaily dressed visitors," and gently mocking her desire to show off her "new silk dress and flounces" (vol. 1, 207).

While Alice's eagerness to display her finery is excused in part by her youth and high-spirited gaiety, the novel also represents this impulse as potentially damaging—and inherently feminine. In fact, Barbara suggests that women cannot help but rival one another in the acquisition of new and costly clothing, asking

[i]s it in human nature to allow our friends to wear the grandest dresses at balls, assemblies, and—church? Is Mrs. Butcher, the wife of the great meat-salesman, in Leadenhall Market, to have a greater change of flounced robes than Mrs. Taxes, whose husband is in Somerset House? NEVER! (vol. 1, 210)

The narrative emphasizes that, as well as readily flaunting their clothing, women keenly observe fashion. When, for example, Alice Tresdaile becomes the subject of the male gaze as she walks along the pier, she "proudly" and publicly diverts her attention to "the sea and the sunset, and the ladies' fine dresses" (vol. 1, 208). In turn, Barbara's own interest is piqued by a "fine dress, containing within it a fine young lady," which "rustled past [them] twice, and drew [their] attention in its direction" (vol. 1, 208–9).

Far more meaningful, perhaps, than the enquiring gaze of "the dandies and their cross fire of stares" (vol. 1, 207) are the intriguing dynamics of female viewing and display. In her discussion of Victorian women's fashion, Kay Boardman argues that "[w]omen [...] have a profound sense of the constant surveillance of their public selves and this also extends to their surveillance of other women too." She asserts that "[i]n this complex process there was space for women to be the subject of another's gaze as well as to be the subject of their own gaze."[40] This certainly seems to be the case in *Grandmother's Money*, in which Barbara reflects on the "true" reasons for female extravagance:

[s]atirical men in the papers assert that we dress for the gentlemen; quite the contrary, my dear sirs—we dress for each other! It is not for your blundering eyes, which would see a dress half a dozen times without knowing it again, that we run up, in these hard times, such extravagant bills at our milliners'; it is

for eyes brighter and sharper that the silks and satins, the purple and fine linen, are flaunted—eyes which tell at a glance what is real and what is counterfeit. (vol. 1, 209–10)

Implied here is the belief that only women are equipped to correctly read and interpret sartorial signs. Somewhat paradoxically, however, this ability is presented as both an instinctive and an acquired skill; while the capacity to read clothing is "very natural," this is only the case for those ladies who are "born and bred with critical tastes" (vol. 1, 209). Yet once learned, however, this ability becomes innate; we are told that "all the fair sex have eyes for fine dresses" and that "nothing escapes them" (vol. 1, 209). In this way, then, viewing clothing becomes a gendered act, in which the female gaze always penetrates further, or more deeply, than its male counterpart.

It would be wrong to suppose, however, that women's clothing is always clearly readable; while Barbara Bloyce sees little difficulty in drawing general conclusions about dress and class from the urban scene, she also concedes that "first impressions are deceptive, and to judge by them is not wise" (vol. 1, 220). This warning seems particularly pertinent within the context of Mrs. Ellen Wood's *East Lynne*, published in 1861, a novel which not only anticipates Mrs. Linton's concerns about the "modern" woman but also explores the tensions and contradictions of contemporary female fashion. The novel tells the story of Lady Isabel Vane, a young woman who, despite her noble parentage, is left penniless after the death of her father. Although attracted to Sir Francis Levison, renowned for his ruthless sexual conquests, Isabel marries a local solicitor, Archibald Carlyle. Following an unfortunate misunderstanding of her husband's behavior, Isabel elopes with the dastardly Sir Francis, after which the Carlyles divorce and Archibald marries Barbara Hare, the daughter of the local Justice of the Peace. The novel's dramatic third volume sees the return of Lady Isabel, who, having been abandoned by her lover and disfigured in an accident, returns to her original home, disguised as a middle-aged widow, to act as governess to her own children.

Despite Isabel's damaged moral standing as an adulteress, there is a sense in which she is redeemed by her visual appearance, in terms of both her clothing and aristocratic deportment. Early in the novel, she is commended for her lack of participation in fashionable culture; we learn that she has been somewhat removed from the corrupting influence of fashionable society, having been "reared as an English girl should be, not to frivolity and foppery."[41] Indeed, the moral differences between Mr. Carlyle's first and second wives seem to draw upon the growing polarization between the "traditional" and "modest" young English girl on one hand, and the "modern" woman on the other. To use Mrs. Linton's terms, it would seem that Isabel can be associated with the "old English ideal," while Barbara Hare, who continually seeks to distinguish herself through dress, prefigures the Girl of the Period.

The interplay of female gazes within the novel provides an intriguing commentary on contemporary clothing. This initially becomes apparent during Lady Isabel's first public appearance in the town of West Lynne. This occasion is highly anticipated by its female residents, who seem, in Barbara's words, "bent on out-dressing Lady Isabel" (106). She perceives Isabel's arrival in the area as an opportunity for sartorial display, and, like several other ladies, purchases a new outfit for the occasion. Barbara's ill-judged choice of costume is described from the perspective of Archibald Carlyle's sister, the middle-aged, old-fashioned Miss Corny: "[a]s she and Archibald were leaving their house, they saw something looming up the street, flashing and gleaming in the sun. A pink parasol came first, a pink bonnet and feather came behind it, a grey brocaded dress, and white gloves" (106). Unfortunately, Miss Corny perceives not a fashionable, well-dressed woman but a "little vain idiot" (106). Through her clothing, Barbara has turned herself into a threatening, gorgeous object, provoking ridicule and pity rather than rapt admiration, and exposing how even "respectable" women of the middle classes are not immune to the seductions of fashionable, modern dress.

When Isabel finally appears, her outfit is something of a disappointment, as she wears a plain sprigged muslin dress and a simple straw bonnet (107). Barbara is initially indignant about Lady Isabel's lack of finery, crying out that "she has no silks, and no feathers, and no anything!" and that "[s]he's more plainly dressed than anyone in church!" (107) Ultimately, however, Isabel's dignified simplicity provokes Barbara to reflect shamefully upon her own appearance. By this point, she regrets her choice of a "streaming pink feather," declaring "[w]hat fine jackdaws [Lady Isabel] must think us all!" (108) Inside church, the female gaze is directed upon another of the same sex; we are told that Barbara, "forgetting where she was," cannot resist the temptation of gazing in fascination at Isabel. Although she concludes that Isabel was "very lovely" and that her dress was "certainly that of a lady" (108), the implication is that the urge to gaze—like, perhaps, the urge to display—should be suppressed.

In its detailed accounts of the wearing, display, and interpretation of female dress, the novel implicitly instructs the reader how to recognize and interpret sartorial cues, and also provides an intriguing reflection upon

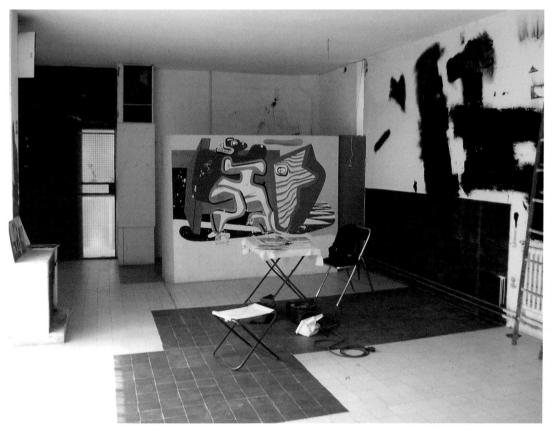

Plate 1 E.1027 living room with Le Corbusier mural. *Photo by Jasmine Rault.*

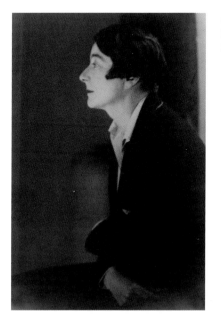

Plate 2 Eileen Gray, photograph by Berenice Abbott, 1926. *Courtesy of the National Museum of Ireland.*

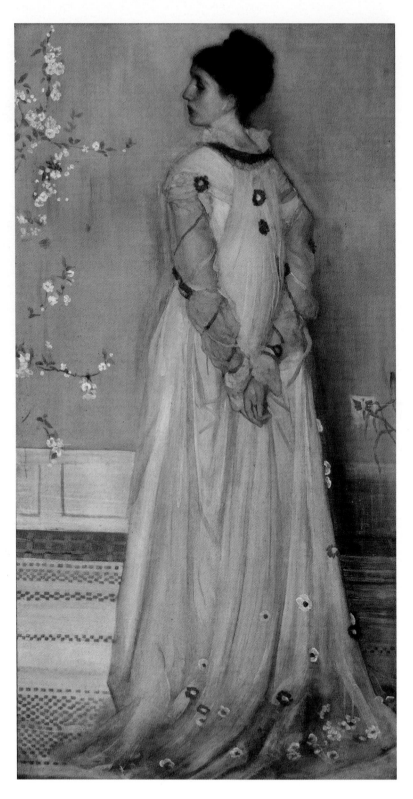

Plate 3 "New Tea-Gown."
Woman's World, vol. 1 (London,
1890). *Courtesy of Queens
University Stauffer Library.*

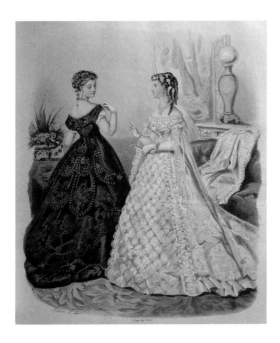

Plate 7 Heloise Leloir
(1820–1873). *La Mode
illustrée*, no. 14 (April 5,
1868). *The Schlesinger
Library, Radcliffe Institute,
Harvard University.*

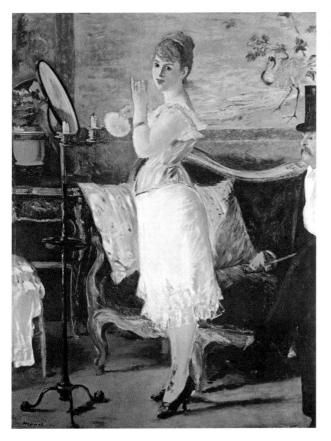

Plate 8 Édouard Manet
(1832–1883). *Nana*, 1877.
Oil on canvas; 154 x 115 cm.
*Kunsthalle, Hamburg, Germany.
Image thanks to Art Renewal
Center® www.artrenewal.org.*

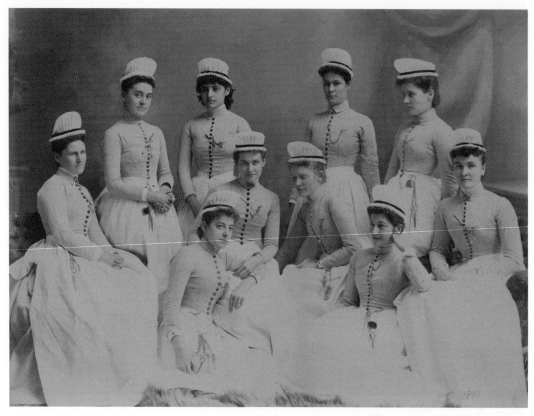

Plate 9 Toronto General Hospital School of Nursing Graduating Class, 1891. *Alumnae Association of the School of Nursing Toronto General Hospital Collection. Photo © Canadian Museum of Civilization, 2004-H0037.8. E2006-00814.*

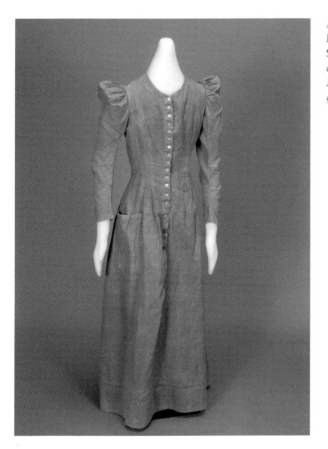

Plate 10 Uniform Dress of
Margaret Elizabeth Lamb,
Saskatchewan, Canada,
ca. 1892. *Photo © Canadian
Museum of Civilization,
982.8.1. D2004–15286.*

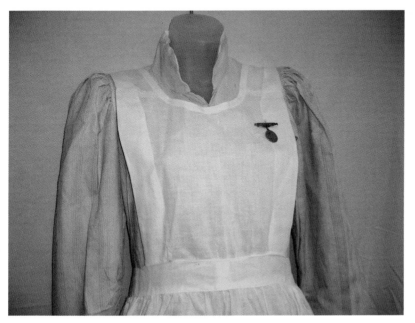

Plate 11 Student Uniform,
Montreal General Hospital,
ca. 1890–1894. *Collection
of the Alumnae Association,
Montreal General Hospital
School of Nursing. Photo
© Canadian Museum of
Civilization, 2009.122,
photo Steven Darby, IMG
2009-0003-0007-Dm.*

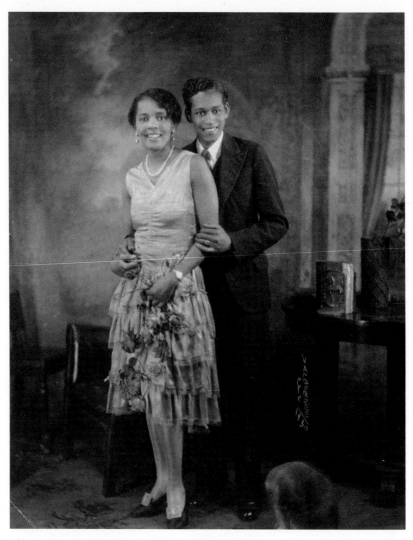

Plate 12 James VanDerZee (1886–1983). *Before the Night Out*, 1930. *Courtesy of Donna Mussenden VanDerZee.*

female morality. Following Archibald Carlyle's first marriage to Lady Isabel, Barbara's bitter disappointment is expressed through her "quieter"
choice of clothing; instead of wearing gaudy silks and feathers, she appears in a simple pink muslin gown. This change is reciprocally reflected
in her "improved" character; we are informed that "[t]he bitterness of
her pain had passed away, leaving all that had been good in her love to
mellow and fertilize her nature" (280). But, while Barbara is capable of
looking both distinguished and restrained, her natural taste leans toward
the ostentatious. Later in the novel, her triumphant, long-hoped-for
marriage to Mr. Carlyle seems to reawaken her taste for extravagantly
modish clothing. The dress she wears for her first meeting with the disguised Lady Isabel, for example, is wryly described as "a marvel of vanity
and prettiness" (495). One contemporary reviewer of the novel, writing
for the *Christian Remembrancer* in 1863, interpreted Barbara's clothing as
symptomatic both of serious character flaws and dubious social prove-
nance. The article, entitled "Our Female Sensation Novelists," draws attention to the character's "vulgar finery," suggesting that she "might be
supposed to be some milliner's apprentice" rather than "an English lady."[42]

The interplay between class distinctions and clothing in the novel is
rich and complex. The character of Afy Hallijohn in particular provides
a fictional or imaginative account of the breakdown of the visual distinctions between women of different social classes. Afy is a working-class
woman who leaves East Lynne in dubious circumstances shortly after the
brutal murder of her father. Although she is believed to have eloped with
the fugitive Dick Hare, Barbara's brother and her father's (assumed) killer,
it transpires that she has secretly spent a period in London as Sir Francis
Levison's mistress. After the breakdown of this clandestine relationship,
she secures a position as lady's-maid to Lady Mount Severn, Isabel's aunt
by marriage, at her grand residence at Castle Marling. Some months later,
when she reappears in the town, apparently to visit her sister, Joyce, at the
Carlyle home, Afy is looking fashionable, bold, and unrepentant: "[t]here
went, sailing up the avenue to East Lynne, a lady one windy afternoon. If
not a lady she was attired as one: a flounced dress, and a stylish shawl, and
a white veil" (381). This description reveals the fragility and instability
both of sartorial signifiers and of contemporary moral descriptors. Afy's
clothing gives few clues about her social status. Thus, in the narrative, a
manservant bows "deferentially" as he opens the door to admit her, assuming that she is a guest of the "lady" rather than a household servant.
Her clothing serves to undermine and disturb the important distinctions
between social categories that were traditionally separate and distinct. The

ambiguity of her position is conveyed through her dress; as Mr. Dill, the solicitors' clerk, points out, "She is not exactly a servant [. . .] she's a lady's-maid; and ladies'-maids dress outrageously fine" (438).

Although Afy is of significantly lower social status than Barbara Hare, the two women attract similar criticisms for their styles of dress. In both cases, clothing seemingly gestures toward the wearer's moral deficiencies, suggesting conceitedness, exhibitionism, and excess. As Afy walks through the town, the narrator observes that she "minced along, in all her vanity" with "her flounces jauntily raised with the other, to the display of her worked petticoat, and her kid boots, the heels several inches high." (593). Like the Girl of the Period, who appeared seven years later, Afy blithely disregards dignity, modesty, and practicality in her eagerness to appear striking and well-dressed. But, Dick Hare, her former suitor, sees Afy not as a lady, but rather, as a woman "dressed up to a caricature" (670). He exclaims, "What a spectacle she had made of herself! I wonder she is not ashamed to go through the streets in such a guise! Indeed, I wonder she shows herself at all" (673). By this point in the novel, Dick, like the reader, has learned to read the moral dangers of boldly fashionable clothing, linking her modish dress with her previous status as a "kept woman." In fact, it is her clothing, rather than her conduct, that he identifies as her primary cause for shame. Barbara, too, is attacked for her style of dress. Shortly before her wedding to Archibald Carlyle, Miss Corny jealously denounces her as "a little conceited minx, as vain as she is high" (428), and as a "fagot," a term which, as Andrew Maunder notes, referred to "butcher's offal" and was "used to designate a prostitute" during his period.[43]

(Re)Viewing the Demimonde

While Miss Corny's comments seem flippant and partly borne of frustration, in the 1860s, the relationship between "modern" fashionable dress and the styles of the demimonde were well documented. As Boardman observes, there was "a fine line between the finery of the lady and the ostentatious vulgarity of the prostitute."[44] In his 1862 *Notes on England*, the philosopher and cultural commentator Hippolyte Taine implies that fashionable English women's clothing was suggestive of prostitution, claiming that "their dress, loud and overcharged with ornament, is that of a woman of easy virtue (*lorette*), or a parvenue," ultimately declaring himself "startled at the spectacle of this paraphenalia [sic] draped on an obviously respectable young woman."[45] Unsurprisingly, this was regarded as problematic, as it meant that visual appearance could no longer be relied upon to denote the moral status of the wearer. But it was not only the

Girl of the Period who desired to imitate the demimondaine, but also more reputable women. In some cases, the dress of noble ladies and that of the high-class prostitute was, supposedly, indistinguishable. In "Costume and its Morals," Mrs. Linton suggests that it was "difficult [. . .] for even a practised eye to distinguish the high-born maiden or matron of Belgravia from the Anonyma who haunt the drive and fill our streets."[46] This similarity, she suggests, is the result of fashionable women carefully scrutinizing the costume and behavior of the courtesan:

[t]he apparent object of modern female dress is to assimilate its wearers as nearly as possible in appearance to women of a certain class—the class to which it was formerly hardly practicable to allude, and yet be intelligible to young ladies; but all that is changed, and the habits and customs of the women of the *demi-monde* are now studied as if they were indeed curious, but exceptionally admirable also, and thus a study unseemly and unprofitable has begotten a spirit of imitation which has achieved a degrading success.[47]

While Mrs. Linton draws attention to the inadequacy of the visual as a method of determining meaning, her article expresses further anxieties about visuality and feminine visibility. Perhaps more problematic than the apparent likeness between "respectable" women and prostitutes is the possibility that, through the reciprocal transaction of viewing, the female gaze itself could be corrupted. For according to Mrs. Linton, the perfect imitation of the dress of the demimondaine depends upon an exchange of glances between the lady and the prostitute. She writes, "Our modest matrons meet," not "to stare the strumpet down," but "to compare notes, to get hints, and to engage in a kind of friendly rivalry—in short, to pay that homage to Vice, and in a very direct way too, which Vice is said formerly to have paid to Virtue."[48] In this way, the female observer misuses her power, using her eyes not to morally defeat the courtesan, but instead to engage her in solidarity by means of a shared, expressive stare. As a result of this, Mrs. Linton identifies a growing, uncomfortable similarity between "Vice" and "Virtue," as the process of sartorial imitation might encourage, excuse, or normalize "fast" or sexually daring conduct. What emerges is a sense of fear that, as Valerie Steele has argued, "not only might girls and women be taken for what they were not, but their actual behavior and character might also denigrate."[49] Too insistent an interrogation of modern clothing might not only betray the "deception" of a woman affecting a different social role, but may also reveal the vulnerability of existing systems of visual signification and classification, as traditionally understood social and moral boundaries became increasingly complex and unstable.

Despite Mrs. Linton's fears, a postscriptum of hope for the "modern" woman is presented in the writings of Mrs. Lucia Gilbert Calhoun, an American journalist who responded to the "Girl of the Period" articles with a work entitled *Modern Women and What is Said of Them* in 1868. Although Mrs. Calhoun unequivocally claims that "[s]omething, clearly, is wrong with fashionable women," who "find in extravagance of living and a vulgar costliness of dress their only expression of a vague desire for the beauty and elegance of life,"[50] she does not perceive the situation as a hopeless one. Rather, we are told that she has encountered some "very fashionable girls capable of large sacrifices for love, or kindred, or obedience to some divine voice," but who "have she suggests that these ladies need "only to be taught that there is something better than being very fashionable" (22). She emphasizes, however, that fashionability is not necessarily incompatible with other worthy personal qualities, observing that she has "found very fashionable girls capable of large sacrifices for love, or kindred, or obedience to some divine voice" (22). Such assertions present a wryly progressive perspective on the modern woman that neither depends upon past models of femininity, nor condemns her on the basis of her visual appearance. This view circumvents traditional alignments between "fashionable" and "fast." Instead, through a mediation of costume, fashionable comportment, and education, women may "come gradually into truer relations with each other and with men" (23). In this formulation, we catch a glimpse of a new, progressive vision of modern femininity, which allows both a moral—and a visual—space for the well-dressed woman.

Notes

1. My thanks are due to Patrick Offenstadt for his kind help in confirming the date of this painting, and for our invaluable conversations on Jean Béraud. The painting is reproduced in Patrick Offenstadt, *Jean Béraud 1849–1935. The Belle Époque: A Dream of Times Gone By* (Köln: Taschen, 1999), 129.

2. Kate Flint, *The Victorians and the Visual Imagination* (Cambridge: Cambridge University Press, 2000), 1.

3. Ibid., 8.

4. Jonathan Crary, *Techniques of the Observer: On Vision and Modernity in the Nineteenth Century* (Cambridge, MA: MIT Press, 1992), 23. Throughout his study, Crary uses the term 'observer' rather than spectator, for what he describes as etymological reasons (5–6).

5. Ibid., 9

6. Charles Baudelaire, "The Painter of Modern Life," in *The Painter of Modern Life and Other Essays*, trans. and ed. Jonathan Mayne (London: Phaidon Press, 1965), 10.

7. Ibid., 10.

8. Although the novel was published anonymously, it has since been attributed to the novelist F. W. Robinson. Frederick William Robinson (1830–1901) worked as a drama critic on the *Daily News* during the 1850s and produced over fifty novels. He also took the pseudonym "A Prison Matron" in order to write three works that contributed to prison reform. Robinson frequently created female protagonists and, as in this case, wrote from the narrative perspective of a young woman.

9. *A Manual of Politeness* (Philadelphia: W. Marshall and Co., 1837), 216.

10. Ibid., 216–17.

11. Mrs. [Matilda Maria] Pullan, *Maternal Counsels to a Daughter, Designed to Aid Her in the Care of Her Health, the Improvement of Her Mind, and the Cultivation of Her Heart* (London: Darton and Co., 1855), 137.

12. Mrs. Eliza Lynn Linton, "Costume and its Morals," *Saturday Review*, July 13, 1867, 44.

13. Doris Langley Moore, *Fashion Through Fashion Plates 1771–1970* (London: Ward Lock Limited, 1970), 96.

14. Valerie Steele, *Fashion and Eroticism: Ideals of Feminine Beauty from the Victorian Era to the Jazz Age* (Oxford: Oxford University Press, 1985), 59, 60–61.

15. "Fast Young Ladies," *Punch*, August 18, 1860, 67.

16. "Fast People and Domestic Habits," *Ladies' Newspaper*, November 22, 1862, 34.

17. Mrs. Eliza Lynn Linton, "The Girl of the Period," *Saturday Review*, March 14, 1968, 339–40.

18. Ibid., 340, 339, 339–40.

19. Mrs. Eliza Lynn Linton, "Ideal Women," *Saturday Review*, May 9, 1868, 610.

20. Ibid., 610.

21. Wilkie Collins, *Basil*, ed. Dorothy Goldman (Oxford: Oxford University Press, 1990), 22, 22–23.

22. Ibid., 21.

23. Hilary Fraser, Stephanie Green, and Judith Johnston, *Gender and the Victorian Periodical* (Cambridge: Cambridge University Press, 2003), 22.

24. "The Pallas Billiard Club," *The Girl of the Period Almanack for 1869* (London, 1869), n. pag.

25. The posture of this figure brings to mind the contemporary fashion illustration. As Valerie Steele points out in *Paris Fashion*, nineteenth-century fashion plates usually included two or more figures, which were arranged so as to show the costume from several angles. Valerie Steele, *Paris Fashion: A Cultural History* (Oxford: Berg, 1998), 126.

26. The arrow, horseshoe, and anchor frequently symbolized the traditional themes of hope and love; in *Sentimental Jewellery*, Ann Louise Luthi observes that love brooches often featured "horseshoes, clasped hands, hearts, lovebirds, harps, buckles and lovers' knots." Ann Louise Luthi, *Sentimental Jewellery* (Princes Risborough: Shire, 1998), 33. Arrows and anchors were also associated with sporting activities; in Edith Wharton's fin-de-siècle novel *The Age of Innocence*, May Welland (who, aptly, becomes May Archer following her marriage) is presented with a brooch in the shape of a "diamond-tipped arrow" as a prize for winning

a ladies' archery competition. Edith Wharton, *The Age of Innocence*, ed. Stephen Orgel (Oxford: Oxford University Press, 2006), 175.

27. "The Thetis Yachting Club," *The Girl of the Period Almanack for 1869*, n. pag.

28. Fraser et al, in *Gender and the Victorian Periodical*, suggest, in fact, that the very behavior of the Girl of the Period suggests, "by implication, how properly conducted, 'natural' young women should disport themselves" (22).

29. "The Syren Flirting Club," *The Girl of the Period Almanack* for *1869*, n. pag.

30. "The Atalanta Skating Club," *The Girl of the Period Almanack* for *1869*, n. pag.

31. "In the Editorial Sanctum," *The Girl of the Period Miscellany* 1 (1869): 2.

32. "What is the Girl of the Period For?" *The Girl of the Period Miscellany* 1 (1869): 5.

33. Ibid., 11.

34. Fraser et al, *Gender and the Victorian Period*, 22–24.

35. "Girls Who Work," *The Girl of the Period Miscellany* 1 (1869): 17.

36. "Fashionable Promenades: In Kensington Gardens," *London Society* 2 (August 1862): 172.

37. Anthony Trollope, *Orley Farm*, ed. David Skilton (Oxford: Oxford University Press, 1985), 278. I am grateful to David Skilton for drawing my attention to this example, and for pointing out that the Latin here derives from Ovid, *De arte amandi*, 1.99, and translates as "the ladies come to see and to be seen." It is also interesting that Trollope's observations on the hunting scene directly contrast with Hippolyte Taine's perception of English horsewomen. In his 1862 memoirs, *Notes on England*, he suggests that they are "simple and serious, with not a grain of coquetterie," and that "[t]hey come to the park not to be looked at but to take the air." Hippolyte Taine, *Notes on England*, trans. Edward Hyams (London: Caliban, 1995), 20.

38. *Grandmother's Money*, 3 volumes (London: Hurst and Blackett, 1860). Although the novel was published anonymously, it has since been attributed to the novelist F. W. Robinson.

39. Ibid., vol. 1, 183.

40. Kay Boardman, "'A Material Girl in a Material World': The Fashionable Female Body in Victorian Women's Magazines," *Journal of Victorian Culture* 3 (1998): 98.

41. Ellen Wood, *East Lynne*, ed. Andrew Maunder (Peterborough, ON: Broadview, 2000), 47–48.

42. "Our Female Sensation Novelists," *Christian Remembrancer* 46 (1864), 217.

43. Andrew Maunder, notes to Wood, *East Lynne*, 437.

44. Boardman, "'A Material Girl in a Material World,'" 106.

45. Taine, *Notes on England*, 57.

46. Mrs. Linton, "Costume and its Morals," 44. Here, "Anonyma" refers to an expensively dressed high-class prostitute. Although the term was initially associated with Catherine Walker (or "Skittles"), it was also adopted more generally, to describe a certain kind of courtesan. See, for example, Andrew King, *The London Journal 1845–1883: Periodicals, Production, and Gender* (Aldershot: Ashgate, 2004), 75; and Fergus Linnane, *London: The Wicked City: A Thousand Years of Vice in the Capital* (London: Robson, 2007), 142–43.

47. Mrs. Linton, "Costume and its Morals," 44.

48. Ibid.

49. Steele, *Fashion and Eroticism*, 128.

50. Mrs. Lucia Gilbert Calhoun, "Introduction" in *Modern Women and What is Said of Them. A Reprint of a Series of Articles in the Saturday Review* (New York: J.S. Redfield, 1868). Reprint, The Michigan Historical Reprint Series, University of Michigan Library, n.d., 13–23. This work comprised an introduction by Mrs. Calhoun, which was followed by a reprint of Mrs. Linton's *Saturday Review* series of articles. It is also discussed briefly by Christopher Breward in *The Culture of Fashion: A New History of Fashionable Dress* (Manchester and New York: Manchester University Press, 1995), 146, 161.

Justine De Young

❧ 6

"HOUSEWIFE OR HARLOT"

Art, Fashion, and Morality in the Paris Salon of 1868

"Sous des noms antiques M. Marchal a voulu peindre deux faces de la société moderne, le monde et le demi-monde, la vertu et le vice."
—Ernest Chesneau

Exemplifying the nineteenth-century conception of gender roles as articulated by Pierre-Joseph Proudhon's stark aphorism: "housewife or harlot," Charles-François Marchal's *Pénélope* and *Phryné* were the sensations of the Paris Salon of 1868 (figures 6.1 and 6.2).[1] *Pénélope* and *Phryné* were hailed by critics as one of the great successes—and failures—of that year's exhibition; their immediate notoriety ensured that everyone had an opinion. Marchal's "angel of the house" and "beast of rapacious luxury," to quote one critic, were the focus of a seemingly endless series of caricatures and reviews in the press and provoked tremendous, lively debate about the relationship—or lack thereof—between dress and character.[2] Seen by some to epitomize the *époque*, Marchal's twin paintings provided male critics with an opportunity to weigh in on the appearance and morality of contemporary women in Second Empire Paris. The modern fashion system had brought into crisis the perception of clothing as an intelligible index of social identity or morality;[3] two competing discourses arose in response to this new ambiguity of dress and crystallized in the debate over Marchal's *Pénélope* and *Phryné*. The conservative discourse as articulated by fashion magazines and some art critics argued that while the wide availability of fashion and fashion knowledge may have complicated the perception of class, fashion continued to be linked to morality and character. A more modern discourse as expressed by the critic Jules Castagnary and others asserted that fashion and morality were not so transparent: "a woman at her work table is not necessarily

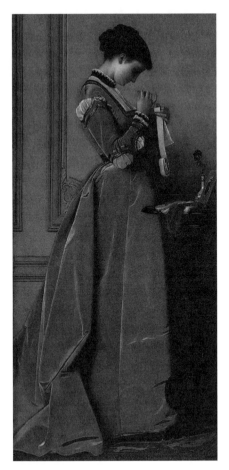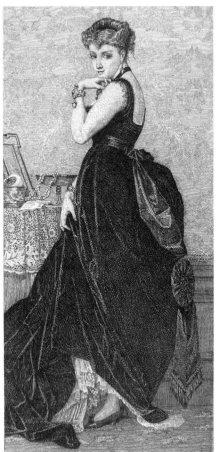

virtuous, however simple her toilette. A woman before her mirror is not necessarily a courtesan, however luxurious her dress."[4] The loss of the indexical power of fashion was particularly troubling at the Salon, where judgments of paintings of modern-life figures had to be made based on appearances alone.

Figure 6.1 Charles-François Marchal (1825–1877). *Pénélope,* Salon of 1868. Oil on canvas; 110.5 x 49.5 cm. *Gift of Mrs. Adolf Obrig, in memory of her husband, 1917 (17.138.2). Image copyright © The Metropolitan Museum of Art / Art Resource, NY.* (Plate 4.)

Figure 6.2 Saro Cucinotta (1830–1871). Engraving after Charles-François Marchal's *Phryné* (Salon of 1868). *L'Artiste* (June 1, 1868). *Watson Library, The Metropolitan Museum of Art.*

Marchal and the Painting of Modern Life

Charles-François Marchal (1825–1877), born in Paris, had made his name at the Salon with picturesque scenes of Alsatian peasant life, which had won medals in 1864 and 1866.[5] Though forgotten today, Marchal's charming, traditional subject matter had made him popular with both the public and critics in the 1860s. In 1868, his shift to the depiction of thoroughly modern *Parisiennes* in *Pénélope* and *Phryné* would catapult him to celebrity. The shift in subject matter surprised many critics, like Marius Chaumelin, who commented approvingly:

Who would have believed him capable of rendering with such delicacy this type ... of the honest woman, [and] with such penetrating insight, this lascivious physiognomy of the prostitute? Mr. Marchal had the good taste, moreover, not to insist too much on the contrast: *Pénélope* does not have the surly air of a dragon of virtue and *Phryné*, at just the right moment, brings back her arm in front of her bare bosom, which partly veils her immodesty.[6]

Marchal's embrace of the fashionable *Parisienne* was part of a larger movement in the 1860s, in which, for the first time, both avant-garde and more conservative academic artists attempted to define contemporary femininity in life-size paintings at the annual Paris Salon. In 1863 Charles Baudelaire in his essay "The Painter of Modern Life" had urged painters to depict modern dress, praising fashion plates and equating fashion with modernity. Baudelaire defined modernity as "the ephemeral, the fugitive, the contingent, the half of art whose other half is the eternal and the immutable."[7] Claude Monet's 1866 painting of his mistress, *Camille*, in a fashionable rented black-and-green striped gown, responded to Baudelaire's call and attracted favorable notice in the Salon. As Monet depicted Camille with her back to the viewer, the painting was pointedly not a portrait, though it, like many avant-garde depictions of anonymous modern women at the Salon, assumed a scale previously reserved for aristocratic portraiture.

Jean Rousseau confirms the wide circulation of Baudelaire's ideas in his review of the new paintings of *modernité* at the 1868 Salon: "*Modernity, nothing is clearer; that is to say, we can paint well nothing other than own époque.*"[8] This interest in contemporary women was due perhaps in part to their newfound prominence in the city; as André Albrespy commented about *Pénélope* and *Phryné*: "This subject is within everyone's reach, and in our time women play too considerable of a role not to attract all eyes."[9] Édouard Manet and Pierre-Auguste Renoir both submitted full-length paintings of women in contemporary dress to the Salon of 1868, but it was Marchal's dual entry of *Pénélope* and *Phryné* that sparked the most discussion and public interest. Marchal's effort differed from that of Manet and the others in that he explicitly set out to define in paint not only the appearance of two contemporary types of women—the bourgeois wife (*Pénélope*) and the high-priced whore (*Phryné*)—but also their moral character. The animated debate over his project hinged on dress, specifically what the "eccentric," ultra-fashionable black dress of *Phryné* and the gray, Renaissance-inspired gown of *Pénélope* did or did not indicate about their morality in this new modern era.

Le Journal illustré credited Marchal with "synthesizing the entire *époque* from both a moral and intellectual point of view."[10] Indeed, writers often saw the paintings as representative of the era; the poet Théodore de Banville hailed them as capturing "All of the spirit of this time / Represented in two volumes."[11] Marchal's pendant paintings exemplified Proudhon's famous formulation of the two possible feminine roles in the nineteenth century—"courtisane ou ménagère," harlot or housewife, just as reactions to the paintings would deconstruct it.[12] The sharp delineation of roles put forward by Proudhon and as painted by Marchal was, of course, not operative in practice or even universally in discourse in the 1860s. Gustave Droz's *Monsieur, Madame et bébé*, published in 1866, advocated love within marriage and encouraged wives to behave as coquettishly as mistresses. By 1884, the book had gone through 121 editions.[13] The perceived collapse of this imaginary dichotomy, which rendered wives indistinguishable from mistresses in both fashion and behavior, was welcomed by some and lamented by others, as will be seen below; however, it was considered by all as characteristic of the period and indeed of *modernité*.

One might have expected that Marchal's carefully designed contrast, elaborated in every detail, would have been accepted by Salon audiences as merely another pair of well-executed, fashionable modern-life figures. For some Salon visitors and critics that was certainly the case, but the wider fascination that *Pénélope* and *Phryné* seem to have evoked from critics, caricaturists, and the public requires further explanation. In an age obsessed with reading appearances for moral truth, when phrenology (the study of the shape of the head to reveal intelligence) and physiognomy (the study and judgment of how a person's outer appearance, primarily the face, reflects their character or personality) were popular, Marchal attempted to create his own physiognomy of sorts, of the virtuous wife and the alluring courtesan.[14] His efforts were perceived in those terms; for example, Pierre Colinot in *Art* writes of *Phryné*: "Her physiognomy is at the same time insolent, sulky and bestial; she is a redhead, of course."[15] This classificatory zeal of the Parisian population must be seen in the context of a growing anxiety over the ambiguity of appearances and their meaning. For example, one critic wrote of the extreme difficulty of discerning the difference between a woman merely walking on the street and a streetwalker: "Marchal had here too great an ambition: he has forgotten that every day we are confounded on the street between the beautiful woman who is merely passing through and the one who lives there."[16]

The rise of the department store and the advent of mass-produced clothing made new, fashionable dresses more affordable and accessible to stylish *Parisiennes*. The leading *couturier* of the time, Charles Frederick Worth, dressed not only the aristocratic court, but also actresses and courtesans. Dress was no longer a reliable index of status, which prompted confusion and ambivalence among contemporary writers that is evident in critics' reactions to *Pénélope* and *Phryné*. Margaret Beetham articulates well this tension:

> The instability of the meaning of fashion generated an anxiety which was not confined to the ladies' papers. Their construction of a femininity which could be read from its surface threatened once again the whole discourse of the domestic woman and of moral management. This threat was dramatically evident because Worth's extravagant costumes were designed and worn by the Parisian demimonde as well as the court. Instead of providing a sophisticated code for distinguishing between ladies, fashion had collapsed that most fundamental divide. Extravagant dress and the presentation of the self as spectacle had become the signifiers of both the lady and the prostitute.[17]

This collapse of sartorial signs did not, however, prevent people from still trying to read moral truth in physiognomy and in fashion; in fact, it privileged the keen and carefully trained eye of the critic.

Indeed, *Pénélope* and *Phryné* seem to have succeeded among critics particularly because they appealed to critics' ability to read clues and master-

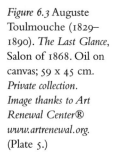

Figure 6.3 Auguste Toulmouche (1829–1890). *The Last Glance*, Salon of 1868. Oil on canvas; 59 x 45 cm. *Private collection. Image thanks to Art Renewal Center® www.artrenewal.org.* (Plate 5.)

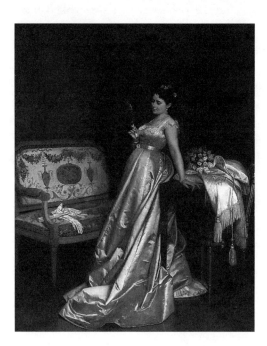

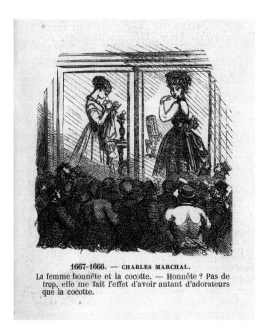

Figure 6.4 Cham [Amédée de Noé] (1818–1879). "Salon de 1868," *Charivari* (May 10, 1868). *Typ 815.32.2750 F,* Houghton Library, Harvard University.

fully interpret them for their audience. Escoffier in *Le Journal illustré* argued that *Pénélope* and *Phryné*'s semiotic ambiguity—and their resulting openness to interpretation—was the source of the paintings' popularity in the press and with the public.[18] The works represented an ideal challenge to the critic's powers of detection and discernment. Reviewers seem to glory in obsessively cataloguing the two works, carefully detailing the women's attractions, in a way they do not those of similar works by Alfred Stevens or Auguste Toulmouche (figure 6.3); *Pénélope* and *Phryné*'s classical pretensions, more ambitious scale, and allegorical antithesis seem to have made the works acceptable objects of masculine scrutiny. Indeed, caricatures of spectators and crowds around the two paintings exclusively depict men, though the works surely attracted a large female audience as well (figure 6.4). This is another important difference from similar genre works by artists like Toulmouche, whose paintings were often shown in caricature with crowds of women around them and were rarely remarked on by critics—feminine interest in the works apparently signified their marginality and superficiality.[19] Marchal's paintings were treated differently—as a challenge of identification and critique worthy of the (male) critic.

The Paris Salon of 1868

The annual Paris Salon provided artists the occasion to exhibit their recent work to a wide audience. The Salon of 1868 filled the Palais de l'Industrie on the Champs-Elysées with 4,213 works of art, of which 2,587 were paintings, 801 drawings and 496 sculptures. Running from May to August, this popular entertainment was attended by hundreds of thousands of Parisians each year; paid public attendance often reached 10,000 per day and was even higher on Sundays, when admission was free.[20] Even those Parisians who never visited the Salon could not entirely avoid it as it dominated the press for weeks. In 1868, 135 critics published at least one article reviewing the Salon, and many published many more; daily papers like *Le Temps* and *Le Moniteur universel* would often dedicate more than a dozen articles to Salon criticism.[21] This criticism allows us insight into the prevalent tastes and opinions of the period from a variety of (masculine) viewpoints. Notably, not all Salon criticism was written; caricature of the Salon was, by the 1860s, a routinized visual discourse and form of art criticism. Marchal's sensual *Phryné* in her black velvet gown and the more demure *Pénélope* were caricatured fifteen times, making them the most famous and frequently caricatured works in the Salon of 1868, alongside Gustave Courbet's contentious *Charity of a Beggar at Ornans*. They were the only works caricatured more than ten times.[22]

Not merely the cultural event of the season, the Salon should be seen as the convergence of political, economic, social, and aesthetic forces.[23] The Salon was a juried exhibition that was influenced by the politics and policies of the government; artists could win official recognition by being awarded a medal or by having their work purchased by the state. Significantly, the state valued artworks differently; the hierarchy established by the Beaux-Arts administration considered mythological or "history" painting the highest form of art, followed by genre painting (scenes of everyday life), portraits, landscapes, and, finally, still lifes. As was much lamented in the press, Marchal's pair of genre paintings did not win a medal; though it should be pointed out that in 1868, for the first time in the Salon's two-hundred-year history, a genre painting won the Grand Medal of Honor, demonstrating the increased interest in and acceptance of depictions of modern life.[24]

Bought for 28,000 francs the day the Salon opened, *Pénélope* and *Phryné* were a career-making financial and popular success for Marchal.[25] This was a huge sum at a time when the fashionable William Adolphe Bouguereau sold major recent pictures for 4,000 francs and the largest history paintings were bought by the state for 10,000 francs.[26] The outrageous sale price, highlighted in reviews, heightened interest even further in *Pénélope* and *Phryné*, which attracted large crowds of spectators; one reviewer claimed the throng around the two paintings was three deep.[27]

This crush of onlookers points to the social aspect of the Salon, where people of all classes would mingle, particularly around popular or controversial artworks. The Salon was a place to see and be seen; writers would often remark on the behavior of Salon visitors and use the opportunity presented by modern life scenes such as Marchal's to comment on contemporary mores and to police accepted norms.

At the Salon, a detailed set of standards and expectations governed critics' reactions and sought to dictate to artists how and what to paint. By violating those norms, avant-garde artists like Courbet and Manet sometimes found their art rejected and, even when accepted by the Salon jury, they were often heavily criticized in the press not only for their unorthodox subjects, but also for their way of painting them. This was true of Courbet's *Charity of a Beggar at Ornans*, whose lowly subject matter and loose brushwork particularly attracted critics' ire. In terms of technique, Marchal's careful academic style and the polished decorative aspect of his paintings could not have been more different from Courbet's. The detailed and refined surface of *Pénélope* and *Phryné* made them attractive to conservative critics and the public—even reviewers who disliked the paintings praised Marchal's technique.[28] *Phryné* (and to a lesser extent *Pénélope*) attracted notice equivalent to that of modernist painters like Courbet and Manet because, like avant-garde works, they violated accepted academic conventions of painting, which expected genre scenes to be self-contained, to be legible, and to obey the hierarchy of genres in their scale (that is, genre works should be small).[29] *Phryné* in her direct address of the viewer implicated the audience in the work, violating the first convention, and Marchal's pendants assumed a scale larger than was expected of genre works in contradiction to the last. Moreover, while Marchal aimed at legibility as genre conventions dictated, as we will see, critics were not always convinced by his efforts.

Pénélope *and* Phryné: Classical Archetypes of Virtue and Vice

While the subject of *Pénélope* and *Phryné* may seem obvious—a demure housewife and a sexy *Parisienne* in contemporary domestic interiors—Marchal aspired to more in titling the works *Pénélope* and *Phryné*. This sort of subject matter was a departure for Marchal, who was more typically known for his sentimental Alsatian genre scenes, such as *The Marketplace for Servants*, which won a medal in the 1864 Salon.[30] Unlike other successful genre painters of modern women, like Toulmouche (figure 6.3), Marchal gave his first paintings of contemporary Parisians mythological titles and a scale closer to that of history paintings. As a student of the academic history painter Michel Martin Drolling, who taught at the national École des Beaux-Arts, Marchal would have been familiar with the myths of classical antiquity, including that of the now obscure, but then popular, *Phryné*.

Phryné was a fourth-century BCE Greek *hetaera* (courtesan) famed for her beauty. As the alleged muse and model for the celebrated Greek painter Apelles and sculptor Praxiteles, she became a favored subject for neoclassical and academic artists in the nineteenth century.[31] The most famous story about her surrounds her trial for profaning the Eleusinian mysteries—secret initiation rites for the cult of Demeter and Persephone. Apparently when the trial for sacrilege was going poorly, Phryné's lawyer, Hypereides, tore open her robe to display her breasts, after which the judges, overawed by her beauty, which was seen as a mark of divine favor, promptly acquitted her.[32] Jean-Léon Gérôme, the highly successful Orientalist and academic painter of antiquity, depicted this famous scene for the 1861 Salon, where it was well received (figure 6.5). He also included the painting in the 1867 Exposition Universelle in Paris, where Marchal likely saw it. The critic Thoré-Bürger commented that Gérôme—and his *Phryné* in particular—was among the most talked about artists in the Exposition, where he was represented by more than a dozen works.[33] While Gérôme's painting of *Phryné* was only one of many in the nineteenth century, Marchal was the first to cast *Phryné* as a modern courtesan in fashionable dress.[34]

If *Phryné* had appeared alone, Marchal's title could have been read as merely a mythic pseudonym for a specific contemporary courtesan, like that of Manet's *Olympia*, which had scandalized the Parisian public three years earlier. By pairing *Phryné* with *Pénélope*, however, Marchal created a deliberate contrast between two antique archetypes of virtue and vice. If *Phryné* was the archetypal classical courtesan, *Pénélope* was the classical model of conjugal and domestic virtue—an antithesis Marchal attempted to cast in contemporary terms. In Homer's *Odyssey*, Penelope was the faithful wife of Odysseus, who left her for twenty years to fight in the Trojan War. She famously remained chaste and fended off more than one hundred suitors by various delaying tactics—among them, saying she would remarry when she finished weaving a burial shroud for Odysseus's elderly father Laertes, which each night she unpicked to begin anew the next day.[35]

In Marchal's updating, *Pénélope* is appropriately engrossed in the domestic sphere, while *Phryné* prepares to leave it for an evening engagement, perhaps hinted at by the letter—adorned with the insignia of a

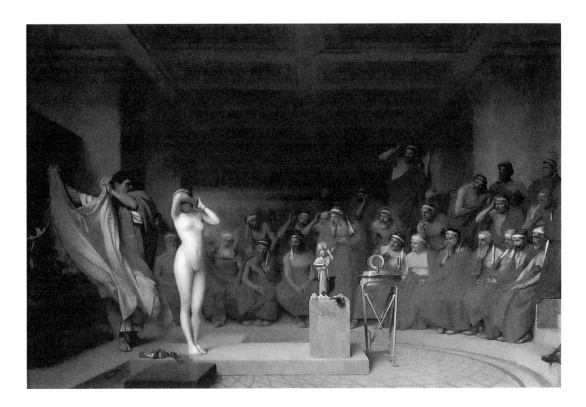

Figure 6.5 Jean-Léon Gérôme (1824–1904). *Phryné before the Areopagus*, 1861. Oil on canvas; 80 x 128 cm. *Kunsthalle, Hamburg, Germany. Image thanks to Art Renewal Center® www.artrenewal.org.* (Plate 6.)

count—on her dressing table. *Pénélope* embroiders intently, working to beautify her home, her eyes focused on the cloth in her hands, while skeins of yellow and red thread spill off the small table before her. On the table rest a turquoise frame with a male portrait image and a white porcelain vase holding a single pansy stem, both of which seem meant to evoke an absent husband. In the nineteenth century, pansies were seen as a symbol of an absent loved one and of the loving thoughts and memories they might elicit.[36] The modest simplicity of *Pénélope*'s table stands in contrast to that of *Phryné*, covered with a fine lace cloth and topped with a large golden bowl, out of which strands of pearls—not skeins of thread—overflow. A gold wedding band is *Pénélope*'s only ornament, in contrast to the heavy and elaborate jewelry worn by *Phryné*.

Dressing Pénélope *and* Phryné: *Fashion and Morality*

Valentine de Kervack commented in 1864 "more than ever fashion is queen;" other writers in the period perceived a shift not only in fashion's importance, but also in its emphasis.[37] What was seen as the previous uniformity of style and slow pace of fashion gave way to a celebration of variety and individuality: "variety is substituted for uniformity, next fantasy has come to pave the road to eccentricity."[38] To keep up with the burgeoning interest and changes in fashion, the feminine illustrated press underwent a massive proliferation in the second half of the nineteenth century.[39] During the Second Empire, not just the number of fashion journals but also their circulation attained new heights. For example, *La Mode illustrée*, the leading women's journal of the time, had 58,000 subscribers in 1866—ten times the circulation of its 1840s counterpart and equal to that of the popular bourgeois journal *Le Figaro*—which is a clear indication of the expanding audience and market for fashion and fashion knowledge.[40] To adapt to the new female readership, *Le Petit journal* and other leading Parisian papers like *Le Petit Parisien* and *Le Figaro* added fashion supplements during this period.[41]

When examining the toilettes chosen by Marchal for *Pénélope* and *Phryné*, it is important to remember that in the 1860s the idea that how one dressed revealed one's character and morality had wide currency. *Excentricité* became a frequent criticism of avant-garde fashions and the women who wore them. In keeping with the belief that clothing was a key to character, Marchal dressed *Pénélope* in an elegant dove gray satin gown with Renaissance-style slashed sleeves. The silhouette is contemporary, but the style is deliberately historic; *Pénélope*'s interiority allied with her more demure gray dress helps create the impression that she is a sober-minded wife who does not chase after all the latest fashions. Yet Marchal's attempt at contrast rang false to more than one critic; for example, André Albrespy considered *Pénélope*'s elegance atypical of French matrons: "It is certain that this elegance was necessary, because if *Pénélope* had the severity of costume of most of the French Pénélopes, she would have been respected as a holy matron and left to her own devices."[42] Moreover, Albrespy imputed a vanity to Marchal's *Pénélope* that he believed to be dangerous:

I suspect that this young woman thought that her dress was perhaps not sufficiently attractive to retain her husband. She dreams of imitating that of the Phrynés, which always obtains the greatest success and is adopted by so many women of the world, that they confuse themselves with them. After the plumage comes the song, and family life has suffered an attack that will take a long time to repair if one is not on guard against it.[43]

In Albrespy's view, dressing fashionably or provocatively like *Phryné* threatened a woman's moral character and French family life.

Despite the doubts about *Pénélope*'s character, which will be discussed further below, her conservatively styled gown is nonetheless in sharp distinction to that of *Phryné*, which reflects the absolute latest in contemporary fashion, as many critics emphasized. For example, the critic from *L'Illustration* writes: "a robe of gray silk is sufficient to dress the industrious spouse; there is virtue in her elegance. *Phryné* is not satisfied to be so economical; she requires sumptuous velvets, perfectly coiffed hair, all the eccentricities of the toilette."[44] Even the contrast in fabrics points to the women's character; the black velvet fabric and ample volume of *Phryné*'s dress was judged appropriate to her role as a courtesan, marking her as particularly sensual with its lush tactile quality and ample curves. Where *Pénélope* is covered up, *Phryné* is boldly exposed—from her fleshy arms and unusually bare back to her low-cut bodice and playfully exhibited foot.

Moreover, in 1868, black had only recently become a fashionable color for evening wear in Paris; in fact, only two black evening dresses had appeared in *La Mode illustrée* in the 1860s prior to *Phryné*'s debut at the Salon, and none earlier than six months before. The close dialogue between Marchal's paintings and the conventions of contemporary fashion illustration is evident in the shared gesture—adjusting the shoulder strap of her dress—of *Phryné* and the black-clad fashion plate model (figure 6.6).

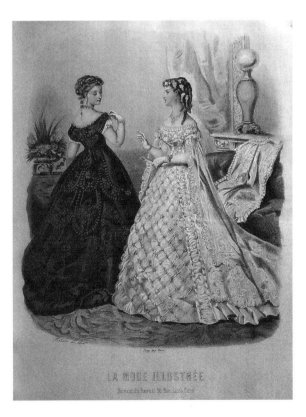

Figure 6.6 Heloise Leloir (1820–1873). *La Mode illustrée*, no. 14 (April 5, 1868). *The Schlesinger Library, Radcliffe Institute, Harvard University.* (Plate 7.)

Prior to this in the 1860s, black was proscribed for evening dress, as the editor of *La Mode illustrée* repeatedly makes clear: "As for wearing a black dress, however beautiful the fabric, at night, with décolletage, one must not think of it: the moment an evening requires décolletage, it rigorously excludes black dresses."[45] The predominant mode of the time was for white evening wear; white and brighter colors were considered more appropriate for evening both to signal a break from the dark-hued dresses favored during the day and because black gowns were still considered rather too funereal for evening.[46] Not only was the color of *Phryné*'s dress a new one, but the style of the gown itself was of the moment; it is fashionably cinched by a wide belt with an elaborate *noeud* (knot) at the back.[47]

Phryné's position at the cutting edge of fashionability was in keeping with her status as a *cocotte* (courtesan), who was expected to follow the latest fashions. During the Second Empire, fashion trendsetting was not limited to the court; actresses and famous courtesans are thought to have helped popularize many fashions with the wider bourgeoisie. This view of the evolution of fashion and how new clothing styles were adopted appears to have been well accepted even at the time, if an offhand remark by Raymond is any indication: "A fashion, which is up to now adopted only by several actresses, who are charged with familiarizing the female public about all the eccentricities of the toilette . . ."[48] Notably, that last phrase, "les excentricités de la toilette," is the exact same as that used by the critic from *L'Illustration* above to describe *Phryné*.[49]

Marchal, perhaps realizing that clothing—no matter how bare or eccentric—was too ambiguous a signifier, added to *Phryné*'s eccentric toilette an additional provocation: her deliberately exposed foot. A deliberately exposed foot recurs in imagery of contemporary prostitutes; see, for example, an 1860s drawing by Constantin Guys, which depicts a black-clad woman meeting with a top-hatted gentleman on a shadowy street corner.[50] Her face is turned toward the man in the scene, but with her right hand she lifts the hem of her skirt, thus exposing her *bottines* and a bit of leg. While women were lifting their skirts and revealing their petticoats daily indoors and out, the deliberate provocation of posing in such a manner and *Phryné*'s exposing her shoe and stocking without obvious reason and in a painting is unusual.[51] *L'Illustration*'s critic warned the reader about *Phryné*: "Beware! That high-heeled shoe, that embroidered stocking, hides perhaps the forked foot of a cousin of Satan."[52] Marchal thus relied on *Phryné*'s extravagant black dress and titillating gesture—in contrast to *Pénélope*'s modest dress and interiority—to secure her identification as a courtesan.

Marchal's symbolic aim with *Pénélope* and *Phryné* was ambitious and largely divided critics and caricaturists into two opposed camps: those who accepted his antithesis as perfectly successful and those who dissented, finding the contrast unsatisfying. *L'Illustration*'s critic was among those who accepted Marchal's intended contrast as unproblematic, praising Marchal for having "perfectly succeeded [in depicting] these two opposed types of modern life."[53] Charles Wallut's judgment in the *Musée des familles* is typical of the dozens of critics who praised Marchal's project: "The antithesis is shown in a discreet and correct way. Here, the hardworking spouse in a gray silk gown, with an honest and chaste look, stands before her work-table; there, the courtesan, whose carefully studied toilette heightens her provocative beauty."[54]

Similarly, some caricaturists seized upon the antithesis, exaggerating the contrast Marchal created between *Pénélope* and *Phryné* by overloading the two works with additional symbols. For example, Carlo Gripp on the cover of *L'Image* freed *Pénélope* and *Phryné* from their canvases, casting them as real women at the entrance to the Salon, and gave them additional props to signal their identities, even as their names hover in the air above them (figure 6.7). *Pénélope* gains a pair of spectacles and intently mends a sock, rather than the embroidery in the painting; while *Phryné*, now wearing high-heeled boots, hikes her skirt up to her knee and nonchalantly holds a paper "*cocotte*" over her shoulder. The folded paper *cocotte* was a traditional child's representation of a chicken, but as *cocotte* was also slang for a prostitute, it is employed here to signal *Phryné*'s occupation.[55] In a caricature by André Gill, *Pénélope* is literally self-effacing, the needle she holds so close to her face in the painting has, in the caricature, carved a concave hole in her face (figure 6.8).

For other critics, like Albrespy quoted above, the moral superiority of *Pénélope* was not so self-evident. More than one critic believed that *Pénélope* could also be a courtesan; as one wrote, her "false air of modesty does not impress me at all and thus I do not find the antithesis very convincing."[56] Cham in his caricature of the crowd before *Pénélope* and *Phryné* is similarly skeptical about the dichotomy between *femme honnête* and courtesan that Marchal attempts (figure 6.4). He emphasizes *Phryné*'s sensuality, placing her finger provocatively near her lips, rather than on her shoulder, and has doubled the size of *Pénélope*'s embroidery.[57] The point, however, is not about the difference between the two women, but instead the similar effect they have on men; the caption features one spectator remarking, "The honest woman and the courtesan," to which another

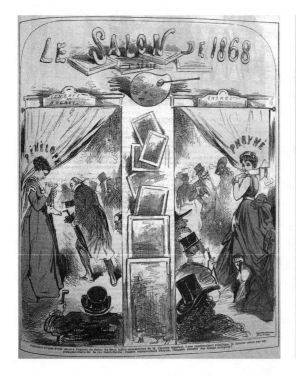

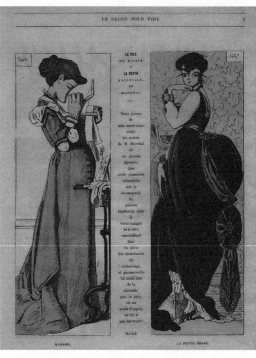

responds, "Honest? Hardly, she seems to have just as many admirers as the courtesan." The crowds around *Pénélope,* like her many suitors in the myth, cast doubt upon her character. Guiffrey in the *Journal des beaux-arts et de la littérature* similarly questioned *Pénélope*'s supposed virtue, declaring that:

If Mr. Marchal wanted to paint two fashion plates, I declare myself completely satisfied. As for a moral opposition, I cannot accept it. This girl, with her bulging waist, is not the honest and pure middle-class woman whom the author calls, I do not know why, Pénélope (didn't he mean Lucretia?). It seems to me that she is cut from same cloth as her neighbor. As for that one, she is admirably in her role; she is truly the *hétaïre* named Phryné; but frankly, nothing justifies the passion of the public for these two women, unless one sees in them one of the signs of our time.[58]

Thus, for some critics, *Pénélope*'s absorption in her embroidery and relatively modest costume could not secure her respectability. While for others, even the extreme and eccentric toilette that Marchal chose for *Phryné*—a bare, black velvet evening gown—and her provocative gesture were not sufficient to mark her as a courtesan.

Before rendering judgment, Grangedor in the *Gazette des Beaux-Arts* first acknowledges the difficulty of the task Marchal has undertaken; that is, to personify "the most disparate feminine types, taken from the elegant world of Paris . . . the ambiguous character of which it is difficult to define and is still more difficult to symbolize."[59] Grangedor does not believe Marchal has succeeded in his attempt, as he does not believe the distinctions Marchal makes are sufficient to distinguish between the two women:

The moral contrast the artist wanted to produce in opposing the reserve of a *Pénélope* with the provocative casualness of a *Phryné* of the demimonde is sadly not sufficiently emphasized: the symmetry of their analogous poses and the identical character of their toilettes—one a morning dress, the other evening—do not sufficiently characterize the profound differences in morality that the painter wished to make evident.[60]

Even Thoré-Bürger, who admired Marchal's antithesis, acknowledged that morality in general had shifted from Homeric times and *Pénélope*'s virtue should perhaps not be trusted: "Between us, I advise Odysseus to return home as soon as possible… as we are no longer in Ithaca and morals have changed since the time of Homer."[61]

Caricaturists often elided the differences between the two paintings, abandoning the cues of fashion and gesture chosen by Marchal and depicting *Pénélope* and *Phryné* instead in the style of contemporary fashion plates. Pitou in *La Marotte* reduces *Pénélope* and *Phryné* to wood mannequins bearing the caption: "Toilette d'hiver [winter]—Toilette d'été [summer]."[62] This treatment eliminated the moral contrast Marchal took such pains to create by making both women simply models for fashionable clothing. Darjou in *L'Eclipse* shows the two women as dolls displayed on stands—their feet dangling in the air—which nullifies the provocation of *Phryné*'s lifted skirt (figure 6.9). They are merely Marchal's "little dolls" standing at identical tables—different only in the color and cut of their dresses. Caricaturists, like critics, thus highlighted the instability and insubstantiality of fashion as a signifier of moral difference. The ready accessibility of fashionable clothing, displayed in department store windows, advertised in fashion plates, and discussed in fashion journals, made the construction of bourgeois femininity accessible to all who could pay, just as the lavish toilettes created by couturiers like Worth were available to the court, but also to the courtesan. Thus, despite Marchal's best efforts, the modernity and ambiguity of fashion resisted his attempts to equate clothing with character. A simple gray dress did not make a woman virtuous and a lavish black toilette—no matter how eccentric—did not make her immoral.

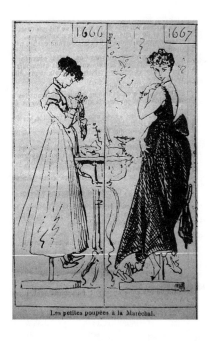

Beyond Marchal: Manet, Fashion, and the Contemporary Courtesan

Pénélope and *Phryné* not only attracted the eyes of critics, caricaturists, poets, and the public, but those of artists as well. Édouard Manet, whose interest in the demimonde was well established by his notorious painting of *Olympia*, seems to have taken an interest in Marchal's 1868 paintings. There is little doubt that Manet would have seen the works in the Salon of 1868. Not only were the paintings among the most famous and most reproduced in the Salon—after all, at least five different engravings and fifteen caricatures were published in virtually every illustrated periodical that covered the Salon—but also, due to their similar last names, Manet and Marchal's paintings would have hung near each other at the exhibition; indeed, their entries in the Salon catalogue were directly across from each other.[63]

The late 1860s marked a shift in Manet's career from drawing inspiration from art of the past—he famously referenced Titian's *Venus of Urbino* in his 1863 *Olympia*—to citing contemporary works.[64] In his 1876 *Nana* (figure 6.10), Manet united the fascination with women's fashion that had defined his work of the late 1860s and 1870s with his early interest in the courtesan in her boudoir, which he had treated to sensational effect in *Olympia*.[65] *Nana*, like *Phryné*, a prostitute with her hair swept up off her neck, stares out at the viewer—her body in profile, but her head turned to the left to confront the spectator's gaze.[66] In contrast to *Phryné*'s heavy black velvet gown, *Nana* stands only in her pale blue corset and the first

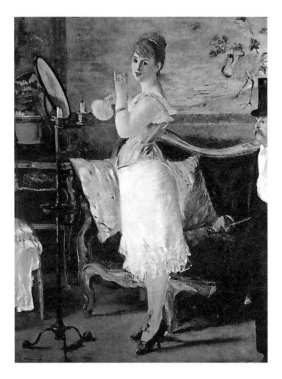

Figure 6.10 Édouard
Manet (1832–1883).
Nana, 1877. Oil on
canvas; 154 x 115 cm.
*Kunsthalle, Hamburg,
Germany. Image thanks
to Art Renewal Center®
www.artrenewal.org.*
(Plate 8.)

of her white petticoats—her blue stockings are visible almost to her
knee, much as *Phryné's* were in caricatures. Manet recognized—perhaps
taking his cues from the reception of Marchal's *Phryné*—that to nail
down securely the identity of a contemporary courtesan in her boudoir
she had to be stripped of her (black) dress. With the advent of modern
fashion, dress had become too unstable a signifier and could easily conceal rather than reveal a woman's moral and social identity. While
Marchal attempted to locate *Phryné* securely in the demimonde through
her dress and deportment, Manet provided not just coy clues to *Nana's*
profession, but an actual client waiting at the painting's edge.[67]

As pendant works, *Pénélope* and *Phryné* permitted Salon visitors to
endlessly compare and contrast them—the wife and the whore—and
they offered Salon critics the opportunity to discuss the physiognomies
of these two "types" of modern women. Modernity and the modern
fashion system had prompted a crisis of identification on the streets of
Paris that was mirrored in reactions to art of the time. Discussion of
painters' depictions of contemporary women brought two competing
discourses of fashion to the fore; while some insisted that nothing had
changed and that fashion continued to be transparent, others found in
modernity a fracturing of art, fashion, gender, and class definitions. *Pénélope* and *Phryné* served as a site for the debate over the transparency of

appearances and their reliability as an index of morality and character. Marchal's *Pénélope* and *Phryné* may not have truly "synthesized the entire époque from a moral and intellectual point of view," as one critic claimed, but they do provide invaluable insight into modern Paris of the 1860s, where the modes and meanings of fashion were constantly shifting and painters and the public struggled to keep up.[68]

Notes

"Under ancient names Mr. Marchal wanted to paint the two faces of modern society, the *monde* and the *demimonde*, virtue and vice." Ernest Chesneau, "Salon de 1868 [June 1868]," *Le Constitutionnel* 164 (June 12, 1868). All translations, unless otherwise noted, are my own.

1. I would like to acknowledge and thank S. Hollis Clayson of Northwestern University for her close, incisive reading of a draft of this essay. Kathryn Calley Galitz and the Nineteenth-Century, Modern and Contemporary Art department at The Metropolitan Museum of Art provided key access and insight, as did Helen Burnham and Emily Banis of the Museum of Fine Arts, Boston. I am grateful also for the invaluable feedback I received on versions of this paper presented at The Metropolitan Museum of Art 2007 Fellows' Symposium and at the Courtauld History of Dress Association's 2007 Conference, "Black and White." Research for this essay, written while a Jane and Morgan Whitney Fellow at the Metropolitan Museum, was also generously supported by a Mellon travel grant from the Alice Kaplan Institute for the Humanities.

2. In discussing the reaction of men before the painting, Cluseret affirmed: "Plus d'un, j'en suis sûr, avait comme moi le respect au cœur en regardant cet ange du foyer trompant l'attente par le travail, et le dégoût sur les lèvres en contemplant cette fauve de la luxure rapace." Gustave Cluseret, "Le Salon [June 1868]," *L'Art*, no. 7 (June 11, 1868): 1.

3. For more on this crisis, see Hollis Clayson, *Painted Love: Prostitution in French Art of the Impressionist Era* (New Haven: Yale University Press, 1991).

4. "Une dame à sa table de travail n'est pas nécessairement une vertu, si simple que soit sa toilette. Une dame devant son miroir n'est pas nécessairement une courtisane, si luxueuse soit sa robe." Jules-Antoine Castagnary, "Beaux-Arts. Salon de 1868," in *Le bilan de l'année 1868, politique, littéraire, dramatique* (Paris: Armand le Chevalier, 1869), 353–54.

5. Victor Fournel, "Charles Marchal," in *Les artistes français contemporains: peintres, sculpteurs* (Tours: Alfred Mame et fils, 1884), 409–16.

6. "Qui l'aurait cru capable de rendre avec tant de délicatesse ce type si fin, si suave, de la femme honnête, avec un accent si pénétrant, cette physionomie lascive de la prostituée? M. Marchal a eu le bon goût, d'ailleurs de ne pas trop insister sur le contraste: *Pénélope* n'a pas l'air revêche d'un dragon de vertu et *Phryné* ramène fort à propos, devant sa gorge nue, un bras qui voile en partie son impudicité." Marius Chaumelin, "Salon de 1868 [originally published in *La Presse*]," in *L'Art contemporain* (Paris: Librairie Renouard, 1873), 127.

7. Charles Baudelaire, *The Painter of Modern Life and Other Essays*, trans. Jonathan Mayne (London: Phaidon, 1964), 13.

8. "La *modernité*, rien de plus clair; cela veut dire que nous ne pouvons bien peindre aucune autre époque que la nôtre. Tout le reste ne peut être qu'hypothèse, convention, source d'erreurs, cause de faux pas sans nombre." Jean Rousseau, "Le Genre et ce qu'on appelle la modernité," *L'Univers illustré*, 701 (June 20, 1868): 383.

9. "Ce sujet est à la portée de tout le monde, et de notre temps la femme joue un rôle trop considérable pour ne pas attirer tous les regards." André Albrespy, "Beaux-Arts. L'Exposition des beaux-arts en 1868," *La Revue chrétienne* 15, no. 8 (August 5, 1868): 469.

10. Henri Escoffier, "Salon de 1868. VII," *Le Journal illustré*, 229 (June 28, 1868): 203.

11. "Toute l'âme de ce temps-ci / Représentée en deux volumes." Théodore de Banville, "Pénélope et Phryné (May 1868)," in *Poésies complètes: odes funambulesques* (Paris: G. Charpentier, 1883).

12. Pierre-Joseph Proudhon, *Système des contradictions Economiques, ou, Philosophie de la misère*, vol. 2 (Paris: Guillaumin et cie, 1846), 197.

13. James F. McMillan, *Housewife or Harlot: The Place of Women in French Society, 1870–1940* (New York: St. Martin's Press, 1981), 35.

14. For more on physiognomy in the period, see Melissa Percival and Graeme Tytler, *Physiognomy in Profile: Lavater's Impact on European Culture* (Newark: University of Delaware Press, 2005). Judith Wechsler, *A Human Comedy: Physiognomy and Caricature in 19th-Century Paris* (Chicago: University of Chicago Press, 1982).

15. "La physionomie est à la fois insolente, boudeuse et bestiale; elle est rousse naturellement." Pierre Colinot, "A travers l'exposition," *L'Art* no. 5 (May 29, 1868): 6.

16. "M. Marchal avait là une prétention trop grande; il a oublié que chaque jour nous confondons sur le trottoir la belle qui ne fait qu'y passer avec celle qui l'habite." Paul Dimpre, "Exposition des beaux-arts," *Le Monde artiste* (July 4, 1868): 2.

17. Margaret Beetham, *A Magazine of Her Own? Domesticity and Desire in the Woman's Magazine, 1800–1914* (London: Routledge, 1996), 105.

18. "Nous avons vu tout cela et bien d'autres choses encore dans les deux tableaux de M. Marchal. Il est certain que le public y a découvert bien des sous-entendus, ceux-là ou d'autres. C'est pour cela qu'il s'est attaché à les proclamer des chefs-d'œuvre." Escoffier, "Salon de 1868. VII," 203.

19. See, for example, Bertall, "Le Magasin des demoiselles," *Journal amusant*, no. 700 (May 29, 1869): 5.

20. Harrison C. White and Cynthia A. White, *Canvases and Careers: Institutional Change in the French Painting World* (Chicago: University of Chicago Press, 1993), 30–31.

21. Christopher Parsons and Martha Ward, *A Bibliography of Salon Criticism in Second Empire Paris* (Cambridge: Cambridge University Press, 1986).

22. Thierry Chabanne, *Les Salons Caricaturaux* (Paris: Réunion des Musées nationaux, 1990), 29–30.

23. I owe this characterization in part to Arden Reed, who described the Salon as an economic, political and aesthetic entity, to which I would add the social. Arden Reed, *Manet, Flaubert, and the Emergence of Modernism: Blurring Genre Boundaries* (Cambridge: Cambridge University Press, 2003), 27.

24. *Bible Reading: Protestant Interior in Alsace*, by the even then obscure Gustave Brion.

25. Charles Blanc, "Salon de 1868," *Le Temps*, no. 2669 (May 26, 1868).

26. For contemporary prices of academic and avant-garde painting, see White and White, cited above, and Stephen Bann, "Reassessing Repetition in Nineteenth-Century Academic Painting: Delaroche, Gérôme, Ingres," in *The Repeating Image: Multiples in French Painting from David to Matisse*, ed. Eik Kahng (Baltimore: Walters Art Museum, 2007).

27. Victor Fournel describes the throngs around Marchal's two moderately sized (110 x 50 cm) canvases: "Il faut percer une triple barrière de spectateurs pour arriver jusqu'à lui." Fournel, "Charles Marchal," 412.

28. Ben Aymed deemed the works: "a banal thought that leaves you cold and moves you not at all," but is quick to qualify that "as for the execution, it is very beautiful." / "une pensée banale qui vous laisse froid et ne vous émeut nullement; comme exécution, c'est très joli, les étoffes sont bien réussies, les physionomies sont finement tracées." Ben Aymed, "Exposition des beaux-arts," *L'Indépendance parisienne*, no. 46 (July 5, 1868): 4.

29. John House, "Manet's Naïveté," *Burlington Magazine* 128, no. 997 (April 1986): 3.

30. "Distribution des récompenses aux artistes exposants du Salon de 1864," *Moniteur du Soir*, July 7, 1864.

31. "Praxiteles," in *The Oxford Classical Dictionary*, ed. Simon Hornblower and Antony Spawforth (Oxford: Oxford University Press, 1996), 1242.

32. Craig Cooper, "Hyperides and the Trial of Phryné," *Phoenix* 49, no. 4 (Winter 1995): 303–18.

33. W. [Théophile Thoré] Bürger, *Salons de W. Bürger, 1861 à 1868* (Paris: Renouard, 1870), 345.

34. For an extensive overview of the iconographical treatment of *Phryné* in nineteenth-century art, see Joachim Heusinger von Waldegg, "Jean-Léon Gérômes 'Phryne vor den richtern,'" in *Jahrbuch der hamburger kunstsammlungen*, vol. 17 (Hamburg: E. Hauswedell, 1972), 122–42.

35. "Penelope," in *The Oxford Classical Dictionary*, ed. Simon Hornblower and Antony Spawforth (Oxford: Oxford University Press, 1996), 1135. See also Homer's *Odyssey* 2.93ff, 19.137ff, 24.128ff.

36. Books on flowers and their meanings, which first appeared in France at the beginning of the nineteenth century, were common by this time. For a comparative study of these books, see Judith Walsh, "The Language of Flowers in Nineteenth-Century American Painting," *Magazine Antiques* (October 1999): 518–27.

37. "Plus que jamais la mode est reine. . . ." Claude Bellanger, *Histoire générale de la presse française* (Paris: Presses Universitaires de France, 1969), 289.

38. "Autrefois la mode avait un incontestable caractère d'unité: telle on voyait une femme, telle on les voyait toutes: la différence existait seulement dans le prix

des étoffes employées; quant à la forme des vêtements, elle était invariablement identique. Tout cela a bien changé; la variété s'est substituée à l'uniformité, puis la fantaisie est venue frayer la route à la excentricité." Emmeline Raymond, "Modes [Dec. 21, 1863]," *La Mode illustrée*, no. 51 (December 21, 1863): 407.

39. Raymond Gaudriault, *La gravure de mode féminine en France* (Paris: Éditions de l'Amateur, 1983), 101.

40. Arch. Nat., F18 295. Bellanger, *Histoire générale de la presse française*, 290. Christophe Charle, *Le siècle de la presse, 1830–1939* (Paris: Seuil, 2004), 107.

41. Bellanger, *Histoire générale de la presse française*, 388.

42. "Il est certain que cette élégance était nécessaire, car si la *Pénélope* avait eu la sévérité de costume de la plus grande partie des Pénélopes de France, elle eût été respectée comme une sainte matrone et laissée à ses occupations." Albrespy, "Beaux-Arts. L'Exposition des beaux-arts en 1868," 469.

43. "Je soupçonne cette jeune femme de réfléchir que son costume n'est peut-être pas assez séduisant pour retenir son mari. Elle songe à imiter celui des Phrynés qui obtient toujours le plus grand succès et si bien adopté par beaucoup de femmes du monde, qu'elles se confondent avec elles. Après le plumage est venu le ramage, et la vie de famille en a reçu une atteinte qui sera bien longue à réparer si l'on n'y prend garde." Ibid.

44. "une robe de soie grise suffit à parer l'épouse laborieuse; il y a de la vertu dans son élégance. *Phryné* n'est pas satisfaite à si bon marché: il lui faut les somptuosités de velours, les artifices d'une coiffure savante, les excentricités de la toilette." S. T., "Salon de 1868. Tableaux reproduits par *L'Illustration*," *L'Illustration* 51, no. 1317 (May 23, 1868): 329.

45. "Quant à porter une robe noire, si belle que soit l'étoffe, le soir, avec un corsage décolleté, il n'y faut pas songer: du moment où la réunion exige un corsage décolleté, elle exclut rigoureusement les robes noires." Emmeline Raymond, "Modes [Nov. 1863]," *La Mode illustrée*, no. 45 (November 9, 1863): 356.

46. Emmeline Raymond, "Modes [Jan. 1868]," *La Mode illustrée*, no. 1 (January 5, 1868): 4.

47. For similar knots, see *La Mode Illustrée* no. 4 (January 26, 1868): 26.

48. "Une mode, qui n'est jusqu'ici adoptée que par quelques actrices, lesquelles se chargent du reste de familiariser le public féminine avec toutes les excentricités de la toilette . . ." Emmeline Raymond, "Modes [Jan. 1865]," *La Mode illustrée*, no. 3 (January 15, 1865): 20.

49. "*Phryné* n'est pas satisfaite à si bon marché: il lui faut les somptuosités de velours, les artifices d'une coiffure savante, les excentricités de la toilette." S. T., "Salon de 1868. Tableaux reproduits par *L'Illustration*," 329.

50. Thanks to Heather Awan for pointing out that in ancient Greek art, an exposed foot or ankle also signaled a loose woman. Artists did not show the ankles of proper Greek women, but free-loving maenads in their abandon often revealed their ankles. For the Guys drawing, see Hazlitt, Gooden & Fox, *Nineteenth Century French Drawings* (London, 1997); or Justine De Young, "Women in Black: Fashion, Modernity and Modernism in Paris, 1860–1890" (PhD dissertation, Northwestern University, 2009) fig. 3.32.

51. Genre paintings of women lifting their hems also enjoyed some popularity at the Salon, though the action was nearly always accidental or somehow

justified in the picture; for example, Gustave De Jonghe painted at least two different paintings of a woman lifting her skirts to avoid a playful kitten, thus exposing her white stocking and black shoe.

52. "mais, prenez garde! ce soulier à haut talon, ce bas brodé, cachent peut-être le pied fourchu d'une cousine de Satan." S.T., "Salon de 1868. Tableaux reproduits par *L'Illustration*," 329.

53. "parfaitement réussi dans ces deux types opposés de la vie moderne." Ibid. A typical dissenting voice, V. Vattier in *Le Nain jaune* concluded the opposite, namely that the two paintings "réalisent nullement l'idéal des deux types annoncés." Valentine Vattier, "Salon de 1868," *Le Nain jaune*, no. 495 (June 5, 1868): 5.

54. "Marchal obtient un succès incontesté avec ses deux figures de *Pénélope* and *Phryné*: l'antithèse s'accuse d'une façon discrète et juste. Ici, l'épouse laborieuse, en robe de soie grise, au regard honnête et chaste, debout devant sa table à ouvrage; là la courtisane, dont la toilette étudiée rehausse la provocante beauté." Charles Wallut, "Chronique du mois. Le Salon de 1868," *Musée des familles* 35 (June 1868): 287.

55. See "Cocotte," in *Dictionnaire de l'Académie française* (Paris: Hachette, 1932).

56. "le type de la Pénélope, en toilette de 1868, me paraît passablement cocotte, son faux air modeste ne m'en impose point et partant je ne trouve plus l'antithèse très juste." Aymed, "Exposition des beaux-arts," 4.

57. Bertall in *Le Journal amusant* features *Phryné* sucking on the tip of her finger. Bertall, "Promenade au Salon de 1868," *Journal amusant*, no. 647 (May 23, 1868): 4.

58. "Si M. Marchal a voulu peindre deux gravures de modes, je me déclare complètement satisfait. Quant à une opposition morale, je ne saurais l'accepter. Cette jeune fille, avec sa taille à crevés, n'est point une honnête et pure bourgeoise que l'auteur appelle, je ne sais pourquoi, Pénélope (n'est-ce point Lucrèce qu'il a voulu dire?) Il me semble qu'il y a en elle l'étoffe de sa voisine. Quant à celle-ci, elle est admirablement dans son rôle; c'est véritablement l'hétaïre du nom de Phryné; mais franchement, rien ne justifie l'engouement du public pour ces deux dames, à moins qu'il ne faille voir là un des signes de notre temps." Jules-Joseph Guiffrey, "Le Salon de Paris," *Journal des beaux-arts et de la littérature*, no. 11 (June 15, 1868).

59. "des types féminins les plus disparates, choisis dans ce monde élégant de Paris ... et dont le caractère ambigu, difficile à définir, est plus difficile encore à symboliser." J. [Jules Joly] Grangedor, "Le Salon de 1868," *Gazette des Beaux-Arts* 25, no. 1 (July 1, 1868): 12.

60. "Le contraste moral que l'artiste a voulu produire en opposant la réserve d'une *Pénélope* à la désinvolture provocante d'une *Phryné* du demi-monde n'est malheureusement point assez accusé: la symétrie de poses analogues et le caractère identique de deux toilettes, l'une du matin, l'autre du soir, ne suffisent point à caractériser les différences profondes dans les mœurs que le peintre a voulu mettre en présence." Ibid.

61. "Entre nous, je conseille à Ulysse de débarquer au plus vite ... Car nous ne sommes plus à Ithaque et les mœurs ont changé depuis Homère." W. [Théophile Thoré] Bürger, "Salon de 1868," in *Salons de W. Bürger, 1861 à 1868*, vol. 2 (Paris: Renouard, 1870), 465.

62. Pitou, *La Marotte*, no. 8 (May 14, 1868): 3.

63. Engravings after *Pénélope* and *Phryné* were published in no less than *L'Artiste*, *L'Illustration*, *L'Univers illustré*, *La Semaine des familles*, *Les Salons: dessins autographes*, *Le Petit Figaro*, and *La Chronique illustrée*.

64. Michael Fried, "Manet's Sources: Aspects of his Art, 1859–1865," *Artforum* 7, no. 7 (March 1969): 57.

65. Though rejected by the Salon jury, *Nana* nonetheless became well known as Manet arranged to exhibit it in the window of Giroux's cosmetics shop on the fashionable Boulevard des Capucines, where according to Huysmans it attracted crowds. Françoise Cachin et al., *Manet, 1832–1883* (New York: Abrams, 1983), 394. *Nana* took her name not from classical antiquity, as had *Olympia* and *Phryné*, but from a character in Emile Zola's naturalist novel *L'Assommoir* (1877). She would later become the focus of an entire novel. Émile Zola, *Nana* (Paris: G. Charpentier, 1880).

66. It is possible *Nana* and *Phryné* share more than just a similarity of pose, appearance, and profession. Manet's model for *Nana* was Henriette Hauser, the mistress of the Prince of Orange, whom Beth Archer Brombert in her biography of Manet asserted was also the model for Marchal's *Phryné*. Adolphe Tabarant, *Manet et ses œuvres*, 2nd ed. (Paris: Gallimard, 1947), 299. Brombert does not seem to know the Marchal painting as she fails to remark on the paintings' similarities and her claim is difficult to evaluate as she provides no evidence in support of it. Beth Archer Brombert, *Edouard Manet: Rebel in a Frock Coat* (Boston: Little Brown, 1996), 384. The identity of Marchal's model is disputed. Phylis Floyd believes *Phryné* bears a striking resemblance to the demimondaine Léontine Massin. Phylis Floyd, "The Puzzle of Olympia," *Nineteenth-Century Art Worldwide* 3 (Spring 2004): note 65. Contemporary critics never identified the model, but instead stressed her universality: "Quant aux Phryné . . . chacun croit reconnaître la sienne." Cluseret, "Le Salon [June 1868]," 1.

67. There has been some speculation that the blue screen with its decorative crane on the rear wall also served as a more discreet sign of Nana's profession, as the French word for crane (*la grue*) was slang for prostitute. Anne Coffin Hanson, *Manet and the Modern Tradition* (New Haven: Yale University Press, 1977), 87, 130. According to Bazire, the top-hatted man was a late addition by Manet—a novel solution to the same difficulty faced by Marchal. Edmond Bazire, *Manet* (Paris: A. Quantin, 1884), 100.

68. "à la grande joie du public, il synthétise toute une époque, au point de vue moral et intellectuel." Escoffier, "Salon de 1868.VII," 203.

III

FASHION AND
THE MATERIALITY
OF GENDER

Christina Bates

🌿 7

"THEIR UNIFORMS ALL ESTHETIC AND ANTISEPTIC"

Fashioning Modern Nursing Identity, 1870–1900

Figure 7.1 is a photograph of the 1891 graduating students of the Toronto General Hospital School of Nursing (TGH). The nurses look relaxed, each striking a different pose, some facing, leaning toward, or touching her neighbor. They wear very similar (although not identical) figure-hugging dresses over corseted torsos, creating the fashionable silhouette of the period. Their dress is augmented by voluminous white aprons and frilly caps, and personalized accessories such as scissors, pens, and pincushion chatelaines, collar brooches, and pocket watches.

This is not our familiar image of nursing. There is barely a hint of the stiffly starched white bibs and winged caps that would become nursing's trademark in the twentieth century. These young women represent the first attempts at the modernization of nursing, which in North America began in the 1870s and had solidified institutionally by the early twentieth century. Historians accept this period as a time of transition in which urbanization and industrialization had so changed society as to create social instabilities leading to reform movements. Massive reform in health care led to the transformation of hospitals from charitable hospices for the poor to socially respectable and therapeutic institutions, a change that depended on a formally trained and disciplined nursing corps. One by one, hospitals opened nurse training schools.

Previously, nursing tasks had been carried out by working-class women, usually mature single or abandoned women, or widows who basically worked as charwomen cleaning wards, watching patients, and practicing nursing techniques they learned on the job in hospitals that were often dingy and chaotic. The new strategy for nursing reform included occupational training for nurses, residential living, and a "modern" uniform

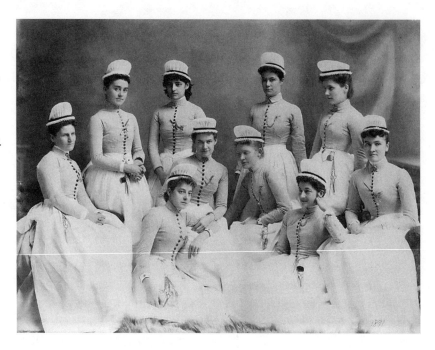

Figure 7.1 Toronto General Hospital School of Nursing Graduating Class, 1891. *Alumnae Association of the School of Nursing Toronto General Hospital Collection. Photo © Canadian Museum of Civilization, 2004-H0037.8. E2006-00814.* (Plate 9.)

that ensured that new young students would look and behave differently from the mature incumbents.

The designs for the first nursing uniforms were varied and experimental, reflecting the uncertainty and ambiguity in creating a semi-professional but subordinate workforce. Nurses' uniforms reveal the construction of a unique ideal of femininity within the masculine structure of the hospital, and enrich our understanding of how gender is manifested, and how it works. Nursing was a virtually all-female occupation, based on the prevailing belief that women were natural to the nursing role. In the hierarchical gender division of labor, the hospital was like a home in which "graduate nurses assumed a subordinate wifely position relative to the male doctor.... Apprenticing nurses were placed in a filial role, as daughters of the doctor/nurse parental team, apprenticing within the hospital much as domestic servants labored as daughters of middle-class households."[1]

The first nursing uniforms followed this domestic model by conflating conventional female fashion with the apron and cap of domestic service. This chapter will describe in detail these often-conflicting modes of dress, and will examine how the uniform intersected with gender, age, and class to both mediate and hinder nursing reform.

Uniforms are revealing artifacts of modernity. They are the public face of an institution, and when they are introduced, or significantly changed, they communicate changes in the functions and values of that institution.

They also operate internally within the organization to create group identity and loyalty. The uniform is not just a symbol, but also an active participant in the formation of institutional and personal *mentalités*. Each day student nurses were physically reminded of the expectations of neatness, cleanliness and personal control when they donned their prescribed dress, pressed their caps, and tied their aprons. As Jennifer Craik observes in *Uniforms Exposed*, "Uniforms are more than just clothing for the body. . . . Rather, uniforms seem to wear the body and produce certain performances."[2]

Uniforms, and images of nurses wearing uniforms, are the salient sources for this chapter. Graduate photographs of nurses are compelling; they confront us with the experience of nurse training at this formative period. The students' expressions, the way they wear their uniforms, their gestures, and their props form a discourse about nursing culture in late-Victorian society. Equally evocative, although in a different way, are the uniforms themselves: their colors, textures, construction, fit, and condition. The methods of visual and material culture studies require us to come face-to-face with the object. An informed but intuitive grasp of its design and what messages that design appears to deliver is the starting point, but of course it is also imperative to take a broader view of the historical and cultural context in which the object was made or used. The close observation of visual and artifactual sources can confirm, inform, or contradict traditional historical interpretation based on written sources. Going back and forth between the object and its context is a powerful heuristic method that brings out new questions and understandings.[3]

Uniforming the "Old-time" Nurses

Among the photographs in the archival collection of the TGH School for Nurses, one image stands apart. It is a faded portrait, taken around 1890, of a late-middle-aged woman, slightly slumped in a chair facing us straight on, with a craggy face, sunken cheeks, heavy eyebrows, and hair severely parted in the middle (figure 7.2). She is wearing the TGH uniform, fitted over a lightly corseted matronly figure, but most compelling are her hands, splayed out over her lap, gnarled, work-worn. She reappears in three TGH staff photographs, standing out in sharp contrast to the more poised younger women.

She is Margaret Davis, who emigrated from Ireland in 1820, and, when widowed, began her trade as a hospital nurse in 1867. When she died in 1905, she had lived and worked at the TGH for thirty-three years. Unlike most of the anonymous nurses who served hospitals before the advent of

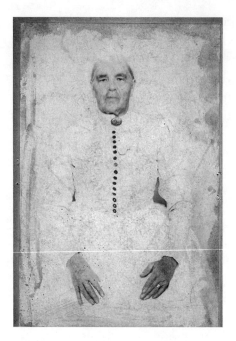

Figure 7.2 Margaret Davis, Toronto General Hospital, ca. 1890. *City of Toronto Archives, Series 1201, Sub Series 5, File 1.*

formal schools, she was lauded in an obituary in the professional journal, *The Canadian Nurse*, as a person "with the kindness of heart under a rough exterior."[4] The fact that the school's alumnae association kept two photographic portraits of her attests to the admiration and affection the school held for her.

This level of respect was unusual; most of the working-class nurses who staffed hospitals before schools of nursing became common in the 1880s and 1890s were much maligned. In order to establish credibility for their reforms, medical authorities would contrast the clean and efficient modern nurse with the "old-time" nurse, raising the specter of the ill-trained, drunken, uncaring Sarah Gamp, a character familiar to most Victorians, created by Charles Dickens in his novel *Martin Chuzzlewit* of 1843–1844. Unlike the modern nurse in her neat uniform, Gamp is slovenly dressed in ill-fitting garments, with a bulky umbrella and enormous hat. Nursing discourse was also critical of the old-time nurses, but it celebrated them if they fit into the new ways—and the new uniforms. Although Mrs. Davis was not formally trained, she was proud of the new school's regime, and "always wore her Nurse's cap and never failed to be present on graduating evening."[5]

Historians have different perspectives on these nurses. Carol Helmstadter maintains that in London (England) hospitals, charges of drunkenness, harsh and unruly behavior, and sexual impropriety were to some degree accurate, not just in nursing, but also in working-class culture in general. In her history of American nursing, Susan Reverby demonstrates how the working-class nurses in American hospitals eschewed "proper" standards of behavior, resisted constraints on their lives and work, and attempted to create their own form of autonomy. Judith Young's study of Canadian pre-training-school nurses dispels many of the derogatory remarks with scant but compelling evidence. Although often perceived as drunken and careless, many lay nurses were actually literate and respectable like Mrs. Davis.[6]

Clearly, Mrs. Davis took pride in wearing the uniform of the school, although she never took the training herself. We get a very real sense of the dilemma faced by these "strong-minded" women on the cusp of nursing reform through the portrait of Mrs. Davis, who slouches unapologetically next to her colleagues.[7]

Mrs. Davis wears the first TGH uniform consisting of a brown-and-white checked cotton dress, cap, and apron, one of the first nursing uniforms in Canada. Even before they had new young recruits, hospitals that wished to present a reformed image dressed their "old-time" nurses in uniform to signal a new era in which the slovenly Sarah Gamps would not do. Indeed, some hospital nurses aspiring to the reform ideal may have created their own uniforms. Consider figure 7.3, an 1881 photograph of

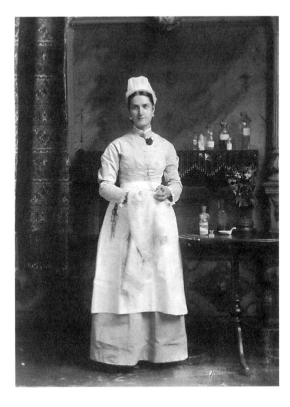

Figure 7.3 Mrs. Miller, Montreal, Quebec, Canada, 1881. ©*McCord Museum, II-61587.1.*

a nurse who joined the Montreal General Hospital (MGH) before a permanent training school was established. Although the dress may have been sanctioned by the nursing school, it appears that there was no set uniform until 1889, when hospital records state "the nurses appeared in their uniforms for the first time."[8] The nurse stands straight, but relaxed, gazing softly outward. She has brought objects related to the practice of nursing, including medicine bottles, a feeding spoon, and a measuring flask she is gently cleaning with a cloth. Other tools of her trade hang from a chatelaine attached to her waistband, including bandage scissors. She is Mrs. Miller, who worked at MGH from 1876 to 1882, when she left to serve as head nurse at the Winnipeg General Hospital (WGH), and eventually won fame for her participation in providing medical services for the Canadian militia during the Riel Rebellion of 1885.[9]

Since there were no graduating classes or class photographs at this time, Mrs. Miller must have wanted to record herself at this initial stage in her career by having her photograph taken in the fashionable Notman and Sandham studio patronized by all of Montreal's anglophone socialites. The format of the photograph was called a "cabinet," and could be produced in such quantity that it could be handed out to friends and family. Right from the start, nurses were aware of the power of the reproducible modern image in establishing credibility for the occupation, a trend that was thoroughly used in graduation and other school portraits.[10]

Unlike the working-class stance of Mrs. Davis, Mrs. Miller is the very model of the modern nurse. Compare their hands: the association of broad, coarse hands with manual labor, and soft, smooth hands with gentility would not have been lost on the Victorian viewer.[11] Mrs. Miller wears a crisp round white cap and a blue print cotton dress, with standing collar and neat white gathered collar band, embellished by a small personal brooch, long sleeves with ruffled white cuff bands, and slight train with polonaise effect at the back. Her apron is so fresh and crisp that we can see the creases. She wears detachable elastic sleeve holders like those used by male clerical workers to raise their sleeves to prevent soiling. This is an unusual appropriation of a masculine white-collar accessory that may indicate her desire to associate with business, as opposed to manual labor workers.

Photographic portraits of workers with the tools of their trade were a familiar genre in the later nineteenth century. Advances in photographic processes made portraits financially feasible for working-class people, and many women laborers including textile workers, dressmakers, and tobacco workers, as well as nurses, chose to picture themselves in their occupational personae. These proud portraits represent the dignity of work, a culture that was apprentice or craft-based, and a working-class mentality. Instead of a parasol, fan, or book, as in fashion plates of the period, Mrs. Miller holds the badges of her trade.[12] She acknowledges nurses' domestic duties in her activity of cleaning a flask, but the medicinal objects represent the seriousness, training, and skill of her position. She has taken extreme care to present a dignified image of herself in her chosen vocation, internalizing the values and beliefs of the reform movement. This photograph is a careful construction of the new nurse, which would presage the reforms and new constructions to come—in ways Mrs. Miller could hardly imagine.

Creating Nursing Identity

Figure 7.4 shows head nurses of the Montreal General Hospital in 1893, with resident medical officer Dr. Hamilton and Lady Superintendent of Nurses Miss Livingston (in black). The nursing school of this hospital was officially inaugurated at a gala event in 1891, attended by Montreal's leading citizens and Lord Stanley, the Governor-General of Canada, and his wife. (Lady Stanley was very interested in nursing reform.) A detailed account of the opening was published by the *Montreal Gazette*, along with lists of staff and rules for the new school. At least a thousand copies were made and distributed. The detailed description of the procession of nurses to the dais is a discourse on the "look" of modern nursing:

So soon as the audience was settled down a rustle was heard at the back of the hall, and the nurses attached to the training school entered in two columns, headed by Miss Quaife, Assistant Superintendent, and Dr. Kirkpatrick, Medical Superintendent. Dressed in pretty pink dresses, with long aprons and neat mob caps, white as the undriven snow, they presented a most attractive appearance, and when they had taken their seats on raised platforms on each side of the hall, made up a picture worthy of an artist's brush. Their fresh complexions, neat attire, and evident enthusiasm for their work at once captivated the audience.[13]

The parade of nurses, their physical presence, their clothing, and their deportment signaled a new era for the Montreal General Hospital to the influential audience. The spectacle was a public relations strategy to put the MGH on the map of modern, reputable, and worthy hospitals in North America. Speaking on behalf of the hospital management, Dr. Craik assured the audience that the nurses' training school would relieve Montreal of the "stigma" of having no trained nurses for the hospital or

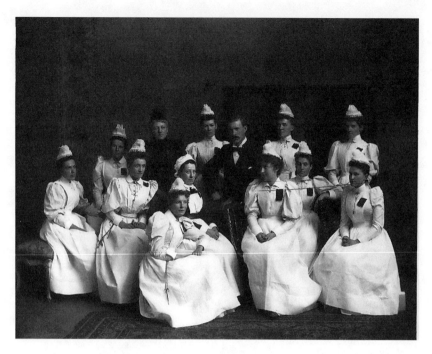

for home care for its middle-class citizens. As a voluntary hospital relying
on donations from the public, he called upon the audience to give money
to get the hospital out of debt, and to support the school. Professionally
trained nurses were needed to assist with innovative procedures and improved patient care. Clearly, modern hospitals needed modern nurses.

The introduction of nurse training schools at MGH and other hospitals created a transformation in the culture of the hospital. Suddenly
there were fresh young faces on the wards and assisting doctors. For the
first decade, these young recruits worked alongside the older nurses, but
soon the latter were phased out. Instead of mature women working for a
wage, therefore, the hospital was staffed by student nurses usually in their
twenties, who, in return for labor on the wards twelve hours a day, six
days a week for two and later three years, received a small stipend, an
education, free tuition, room and board, and a uniform. Once accepted,
a student entered the school on three months' probation. Instruction for
students was haphazard at first, but eventually nurses were able to attend
lectures by doctors in anatomy, physiology, communicable diseases, material medical, medical, surgical, and obstetric nursing. Supervisory nurses
taught nursing ethics and such practices as hygiene, dietetics, and ban-
daging. Once graduated, most nurses left the hospital for marriage or for
work as private-duty nurses in patients' homes. Only a very few stayed on
in supervisory positions in the hospital.[14]

A proprietary uniform was invariably part of the strategy in establishing a new school. While the design for uniforms drew on a limited vocabulary of garments and styles, each school had a distinctive uniform. Graduate nurses who went to work at other hospitals or in private practice often continued to wear the uniform of their alma mater.

How were the choices made about what the first nursing uniforms in Canada should look like? There were few examples of complete female uniforms beyond the prison and other custodial institutions. Were Canadian uniforms influenced by those in Europe that preceded them, or by those in the United States? What do those choices reveal about nursing at this early stage? Without recourse to written explanations, how do we deconstruct this nonverbal discourse? In *Uniforms and Nonuniforms*, sociologist Nathan Joseph defines the uniform as "a social artifact, forming a system of communication which at some level is symbolic of the values, beliefs, emotions of the organization and the wearer." He suggests we analyze uniforms through the rhetorical device of metaphor. Faced with a uniform we must ask: "who [or what] is adopted as the model for the metaphor; who uses the metaphor; to what extent is the model adopted?"[15] Two prevalent models that can be discerned in the uniform: the conventional dress of women, and that of household servants.

"Perfect Fitness of Woman": Fashion, Gender, and the Nurses' Uniform

In order to establish models for the TGH, or any of the first North American uniforms, it is necessary to investigate the significant patterns in the development of its antecedents in Europe. The uniform worn by Mrs. Davis is a descendent of those created in Europe, where reform in nursing originated somewhere in the 1830s to the 1860s, and spread to other parts of the world in the 1870s and 1880s.

The first reform nursing uniforms were created by female Protestant nursing orders. The first was introduced in 1833 at the Kaiserswerth Deaconess Institute's Nurse Training School near Dusseldorf. Its founders, Theodor and Friedericke Fliedner, deliberately chose as their model the traditional dress of a married woman to signal that the Kaiserswerth nurses were to be accorded respect and occupational independence. Strict rules governed the wearing of the uniform: no silk was allowed on dresses or scarves; neckerchiefs had to be made of white linen or cotton to avoid "vanity, complacency or carelessness."[16] In England, revival of Protestant women's religious orders in the mid-nineteenth century included the Sisters of Charity, established by a Quaker, Elizabeth Fry, and an Anglican Deaconess nurse training school, the St. John's House in London. Like at

Kaiserswerth, the uniforms worn by these nurses were based on conventional dress of the time, but were noted for simplicity and lack of ornament. Jewelry and fashionable hairdressing were prohibited.[17]

In her recommendations for nursing uniforms, Florence Nightingale—who had studied the Kaiserswerth and other nursing schools—followed this model of restraint. Invited in 1854 to improve the appalling conditions in the British army hospitals during the Crimean War, she insisted that her nurses wear uniforms of plain gray tweed wrappers for winter and printed cotton for summer, along with check aprons and white caps. When donations in her honor were collected to open, in 1860, the Nightingale School at St. Thomas' Hospital, London, the nurses were issued alpaca wool dresses and print cotton dresses. Nightingale, who was to exert influence over the school, although not to run it, insisted that "no crinolines, polonaises, hair-pads, etc." were to be worn. Later she commented that feminine fashion—"the fidget of silk and of crinoline, the rattling of stays and of shoes"—impeded both the practical movement and quiet atmosphere required for looking after the sick.[18] She deliberately avoided any religious reference in the uniform, as she wanted to put emphasis on nursing, not spiritual mission.

These prototypical nurses' uniforms used the vocabulary of contemporary dress, consisting of garments to be found in any woman's wardrobe. But the relationship with fashion was problematic. Indeed, a discourse of anti-fashion with moral overtones emerges from these first uniforms, a discourse that was widespread in middle-class Victorian society, articulated by the clergy and social reformers. Dress was understood to be the outward expression of inner moral values. Modest dress indicated "harmony, order, self-sacrifice," and extravagance in dress signified "self-indulgence, disorder, and wastefulness."[19] Yet, a complete disdain for fashion could also be negatively viewed as calling attention to oneself, one reason the proposal for pants or bloomers for women was not popularly accepted. Women were to dress in the style of the time, but with simple elegance rather than lavish showiness. Keeping up with the rapid and substantial changes in style throughout the nineteenth century was synonymous with adapting to a rapidly changing society. Fashion was an "outward expression of progressive social values, control, and hierarchy; fashion was a sign of modernity."[20]

The first uniforms worn by nurses in North America adhered to the Nightingale model of restrained convention in female fashion. Initially, two uniforms were issued, following the conventional social practice of changing dress during the day: cotton dresses were worn in the morning for housework and plain wool dresses for afternoon activities, especially

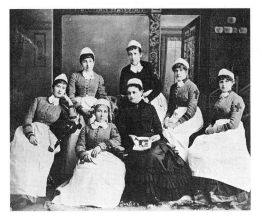
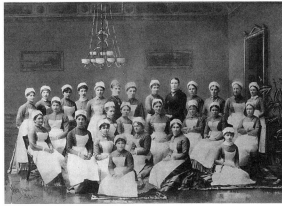

when attending to visitors. In an 1878 photograph of the staff of the
Mack, the first training school in Canada, in St. Catharines, Ontario, the
nurses wear plain dark blue dresses (figure 7.5). They also had blue-and-
white striped cotton uniforms, presumably for morning wear. At the
TGH in the 1870s and early 1880s, the nurses wore brown checked cotton dresses for morning wear and gray woolen serge for afternoon wear.[21]
An 1883 photograph of the staff of the hospital (figure 7.6) clearly shows
the plain woolen front-buttoned uniform, consisting of fitted bodice and
skirt with train. These early Canadian uniforms have the popular shape
of fashionable women's clothes, but are severely plain and unadorned, as
compared with fashionable bodices embellished with inserts or tucks.[22]

Although the double dress code of morning/afternoon, cotton/wool,
light/dark continued into the twentieth century in England, it was abandoned in North America soon after being introduced. At the TGH, for
example, nurses were "supposed to change in the afternoon to a dress
uniform of grey serge ... but this custom was gradually discarded."[23] Portraits of TGH nurses after 1883 show only the cotton dress, so presumably
the wool outfit was already gone by this time.

Eventually, the one-piece cotton dress became the choice for all nurses'
uniforms in Canada and the United States. What was it about this simple
dress that suited nursing in North America? Why was the wool dress
—which had the advantage of being more sturdy and long-lasting—
abandoned? Wool garments were much more difficult to wash, and we
might be tempted to think that a cotton dress that could be made sterile
through frequent washing would be superior. Yet, the idea of uniforms as
barriers to contamination was more a concern of the twentieth century.
Although the relationship between bacteria and disease had been known
since the 1840s, antiseptic and aseptic surgical techniques to prevent
putrefaction were not widely practiced until the 1890s, and had a limited

Figure 7.5 Graduate
Nurses and Probationers,
Mack Training School
for Nurses, St. Catha-
rines, Ontario, Canada,
ca. 1875. *Canadian Nurses
Association Collection.
Photo © Canadian
Museum of Civilization,
2001-H0006.4.
IMG2008-0633-0021-Dm.*

Figure 7.6 Toronto
General Hospital Nurses,
1883. *City of Toronto
Archives, Series 1201,
Sub Series 5, File 4.*

impact on nursing (figure 7.10). Florence Nightingale herself was not accepting of "germ theory," but rather subscribed to the idea that environmental factors such as overcrowding, poor ventilation, and filth created diseases.[24] She cautioned the nurse on the ward to be "ever on the watch, ever on her guard, against want of cleanliness, foul air, want of light, and of warmth."[25] Personal hygiene, however, was more of a moral, rather than medical, imperative to bring credibility and respectability to nursing. It was important for the nurse to look clean, not necessarily to be clean. As Florence Nightingale herself pointed out, it was easier for woolen clothing to look clean and neat than cotton: "better I think avoid washing stuffs, they require endless change to look elegant."[26]

Instead, there were several practical reasons for the adoption of the cotton dress. As hospital staff and students grew in number in the 1880s, it was easier to procure, produce, and inspect one uniform rather than two. Moreover, perhaps the time required for dress change was begrudged by the authorities. As hospitals expanded, laundry facilities were modernized, and it was more feasible to wash the cotton dresses.

In addition to these practical concerns, social conditions in North America were different from those in England. The practice of changing from morning to formal afternoon dress both for household servants and nurses was more applicable to England, where class distinctions were more prominent. The nursing reform system in England codified social differences among students accepted into the first training schools, in which both working-class women and "ladies" became nurses. The ladies, or "specials," did less menial work, and were allowed to have small differences in their uniform.[27] In North America no doubt there were social distinctions among the first nursing recruits, but it was not institutionalized, and all students performed the same tasks (for their level of training), and wore the same uniform.

By the 1890s, all nursing schools in North America required some version of the cotton dress. By this time, new concerns over female fashion turned increasingly from inner states of mind to the body. Medical practitioners, educators, artists, and feminists joined in a crusade to convince women to abandon their highly decorative and artificial forms of dress for the sake of their health. They promoted dress reform garments that were relatively loose and flowing compared with the prevailing heavy and confining fashions. The corset received particular condemnation. Tight lacing of corsets was said to be the cause of a long list of health problems including weakness of the lungs, poor circulation, displacement of internal organs, palpitations of the heart, and even consumption. Since corsets were worn by all classes of women in all types of activities, the dress reform movement rarely advocated disposing of the corset, and instead encouraged the wearing of "health" corsets made of less rigid materials, tightened to the natural, rather than an artificial, body shape.[28]

The first nurses' uniforms maintained the fashionable silhouette created by a corset and the cut of a dress. The graduate nurses in figure 7.1, for example, wear dresses that are almost skintight over their youthful figures, revealing the outline of the corset below. The corset has created the elongated hourglass torso with lifted bust and slightly rounded shoulders, which was in vogue. On closer inspection, however, the constriction of the corset does not appear severe. This is in keeping with advice about corsets from a British nursing journal: "No nurse who wishes to look tidy should go without this often much abused article of feminine attire; but let them be of a soft, pliable make."[29] The concerns of the dress reform movement were within public discourse, and most likely had an effect on how nurses laced up their corsets. But the young women who attended nursing school clearly wanted to adhere to a youthful, shapely figure, which was tolerated as long as their undergarments did not interfere with their work.

The TGH graduate dresses are simple, cut in the "princess" style, with vertical seams from shoulder to hem, without waist seam. This sheath style was popularly worn by middle-class women for morning indoor attire, and was a fashionable alternative to the conventional outfit of fitted basque bodice and draped skirt. Introduced in the late 1870s, the princess fashion was adopted by dress reformers as being healthful because it evenly distributed the weight of the garment over the body. Moreover, while this body-skimming style emphasized the lines of the torso, it did not require tightly laced corsets to give it shape.[30] While no TGH uniform of this period exists, an example of a princess-style uniform from Saskatchewan illustrates the cut and construction (figure 7.7). The front panels extend in one piece from shoulder to hem, with a front opening to mid-thigh level, closed with mother-of-pearl buttons. Two darts on either side of the center front go below the waistline to create the fashionable look of a long torso. One set of darts is cut and pressed flat, ensuring a close fit. The cotton bodice lining is sewn together with the outer fabric at all the seams, a time- and cost-cutting practice for a serviceable garment. The back is not cut princess; rather the lowered and slightly pointed waist seam attaches the gathered skirt to the bodice, creating the dropped and very flat bustle look of the late-1880s polonaise, which nurses could emphasize by tying their voluminous apron strings into exuberant puffs at the back (seen in figure 7.12, and on the nurse on the far left in figure 7.1).

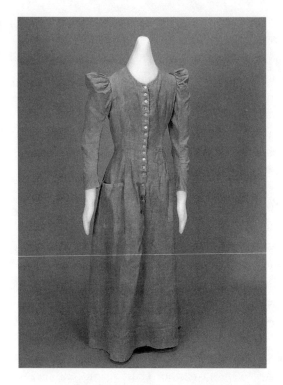

Figure 7.7 Uniform Dress of Margaret Elizabeth Lamb, Saskatchewan, Canada, ca. 1892. *Photo © Canadian Museum of Civilization, 982.8.1. D2004–15286.* (Plate 10.)

The princess style was out of fashion by about 1891, and a couple of years later, TGH caught up with fashion by adding three tucks on either side of the dress button closure, a decorative device that was popular in shirtwaist blouses and basques of the early 1890s (figure 7.8). The most striking change in the bodice was the gigot or leg-of-mutton sleeve, right in fashion, with drooping puff from shoulder to elbow. This voluminous sleeve in all its variations appeared on virtually every nursing uniform in North America.

As exemplified by TGH, the first nursing dresses used styles from conventional women's wear. As women's styles changed, the uniform changed, albeit slightly behind the fashions. Nursing superintendents did not eschew fashion; they allowed their students to follow its dictates by adapting the cut of bodice or sleeve. The image was one of restrained femininity. In their photographs, nurses were posed more like ideal women than occupational workers.

Consider the portrait of two nursing students in figure 7.9. They sit close to each other, gently touching, their expressions dreamy. They wear soft collars with large bows at the neck, gathered bibs, and diminutive caps. The photograph would have been read at the time as a portrait of femininity: gentle, passive, delicate. The reality that nurses had to lift, clean, and restrain patients, dispose of blood and guts, stanch bleeding

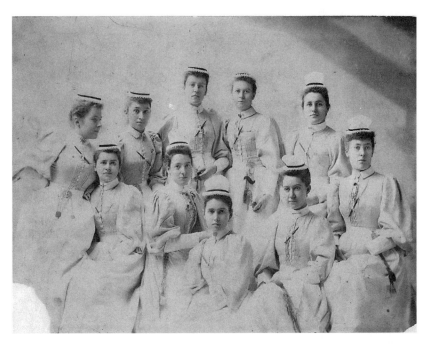

Figure 7.8 Graduating Class, School of Nursing, Toronto General Hospital, 1894. *City of Toronto Archives, Series 1201, Sub Series 1, File 5.*

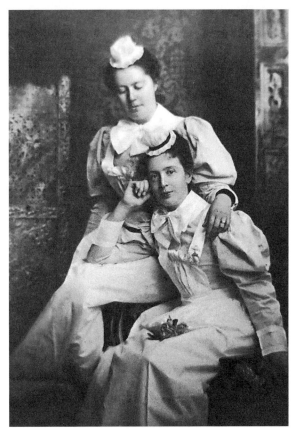

Figure 7.9 Student Nurses at the John H. Stratford Hospital Training School for Nurses, Brantford, Ontario, Canada, 1897. *Canadian Nurses Association/Library and Archives Canada, e002414893.*

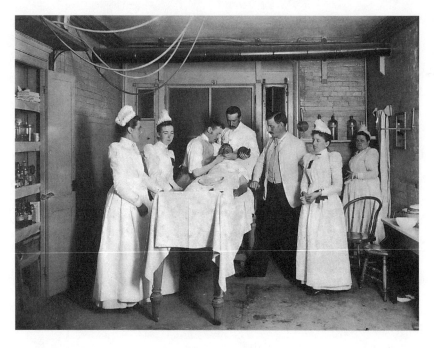

wounds, and scrub bedpans, is not even hinted at in their portraits. Even
photographs of nurses working in the operating theater (figure 7.10)
display charming passivity: the surgeon and interns are busily performing
the work while the nurses are picturesquely standing by, or, as John Berger
says in speaking of paintings of women, "men act and women appear."[31]

The anesthetist and Dr. Hamilton in figure 7.10 wear over their personal vest and trousers the white coats that were provided to MGH residents in 1891. The white coat, as Blumhagen contends, conveyed the
authority of the medical man as a scientist and top professional in the
hospital. The surgeon in figure 7.10 wears a coarse apron tied around his
neck and rolled-up sleeves to absorb bodily fluids but also as a nod to the
emerging understanding of aseptic surgery (although none wear gloves
or masks). For the physicians, their protective clothing aids them in their
expert practice. For the nurses—although they would be responsible for
cleaning the theater and disposing of waste after the operation—their
impractical pink costume, with long sleeves, full skirt, and unstable head-
wear, clearly symbolizes deference to the physician. The whiteness of the
nurses' aprons and bibs was a symbol of respectable servitude, not expertise. The doctors' coats are not a uniform; only nurses, along with lowly
staff such as porters, and elevator and messenger boys, wore uniforms at
MGH.[32]

While some nursing historians maintain that nurses' uniforms and behavior conveyed nurses' asexual status, Kathryn McPherson counters that

"nursing's reliance on both femaleness and sexuality were never completely denied," and that nursing leaders did not repress desire, but, rather, redefined it.[33] The replacement of older matrons with young unmarried women was not lost on hospital medical staff. This is apparent in figure 7.4, where the uniformed nurses with hands demurely folded are arrayed around a swaggering young doctor in his fashionable clothes, who looks rather pleased with his harem of young women. A rare account of the reaction of doctors to the nurses in uniform appears in a local newspaper article about the 1891 MGH nursing school's graduation ceremony, which reported that "medical students testified their interest in the proceedings by frequent outbursts of applause. . . . [The nurses] all were arrayed in the pretty pink costumes . . . the costumes were not the only things that were pretty!"[34]

Nursing uniforms were described by journalists and hospital staff in diminutive and condescending terms such as "neat," "pretty," "becoming," "pleasing." The uniforms both sexualized and infantilized their wearers. MGH Nursing Superintendent Livingston capitalized on the tension between sexual attractiveness and delicate innocence when at a hospital board meeting she brought a young nurse dressed in the outdoor costume (cloak and bonnet) Livingston was trying to get approved. She related that one doctor said that if the cloak were adopted, each nurse would look so "'dangerously nice'" that she would "need a watchdog, an M.D. preferred, to look after them."[35]

Indeed, feminine attractiveness was imposed on nurses almost as a duty. The manual *How to Be a Trained Nurse* advised young women thinking of entering nursing school that "[a] nurse must not lose her taste for artistic and becoming dress because of her profession."[36] Student nurses were at prime marriageable age (20–35 years) and it was accepted that the majority would marry soon after graduation and either give up nursing or practice in private homes when family life permitted. Under the ideology of late-Victorian heterosexual gender roles, women were expected to make themselves available and desirable for the sake of their future marriages and motherhood. The nurses in pretty pink dresses were prime for the marriage market.

Young women entering nursing schools internalized the physical allure of the uniform. Ethel Johns wrote that the first time she put on her WGH uniform, "my reflection in the cracked mirror . . . was dazzling."[37] As a member of the audience at the opening of the MGH nursing school, Jessie Dunlop confessed, "When I saw how nice the nurses all looked in their pink uniforms and starched aprons, I thought it would be a fine thing to be one of them." She was discouraged from doing so because of

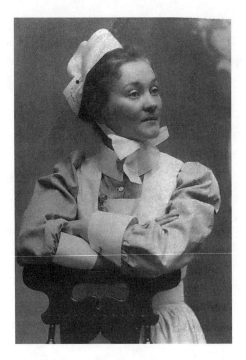

Figure 7.11 Isobel Atkinson, Royal Jubilee Hospital School of Nursing, Victoria, British Columbia, Canada, 1893. *Courtesy of the Royal Jubilee Hospital School of Nursing Archives/Museum.*

"how dirty the place was and overrun by rats." She could not resist the uniform, however, and graduated in 1893.[38]

There were no doubt fissures in this hegemony. Not all nurses wished to be posed as the eternal feminine. Figure 7.11 is a portrait of nursing student Isobel Atkinson of the Royal Jubilee Hospital, who was described in the school's history as a "small, blond, energetic girl." Her posture and expression are quite unusual for this time. She eventually went on to become a superintendent of nursing, and perhaps her pose embodies her future ambitions.[39] She is leaning on a chairback with her arms crossed in a masculine pose. Her uniform is crisp and practical, and her gaze confident, even assertive. The vast difference between this portrait and the Brandon nurses represents a paradox in nursing reform: how do you reconcile womanly tenderness, fragility, and emotionality with the professional requirements of discipline, skill, and physical strength?

This conundrum was addressed by Dr. MacCallum in a speech directed at the student nurses at the MGH inauguration. In the patronizing language common to the many speeches delivered at nursing school inaugurations and graduations, Dr. MacCallum maintained that nursing required the feminine virtues of "sympathy, devotion, and tenderness," and that therefore there is "the perfect fitness of woman" for nursing. The doctor thereby constructed a biological explanation for the innate suitability of women to care for the sick. But in order to carry that argument toward support for the hospital's new nursing school, Dr. MacCallum allowed that, to harness women's natural sympathy toward the requirements of the hospital, "education and training however are necessary to make a nurse."[40] Despite these assurances, nursing superintendents often had to fight for class time for their pupils, as hospital administrators soon realized the monetary savings in deploying their young, strong workforce to work on the wards, and were loath to give time toward their education.[41]

A related problem for hospital nursing reform was how to make it acceptable for young women to enter a realm of male privilege. In his speech, Dr. MacCallum cautioned that "[t]he question of woman's capability to perform much of the world's work, which has been hithertofore performed exclusively by man, has of late years given rise to much controversy."[42] That controversy was resolved by the gender argument that nursing is naturally suited to women, and therefore would not encroach on men's work. In this way, the nursing reform initiated by Florence Nightingale "neutralized this disruptive potential by putting nursing on the public agenda but then firmly tethering the occupation to conventional gender roles, emphasizing nurses' nurturing work, their management of sanitary conditions, and their ability 'to make a hospital a home.'"[43]

The sight of nurses in feminized but modest "pretty pink dresses" mediated the inherent contradictions in the introduction of nursing reform, which was part of a developing ideology of maternal feminism, calling upon women to define a public role for themselves so as to improve society and alleviate suffering. Nursing uniforms appeared during this first wave of feminism. The neat, clean uniforms allied the young women with modern medicine, yet the uniforms' patent femininity adhered to the gender expectations of submissiveness and obedience. When the MGH Board of Governors approved of the school's first uniform, they called it "a composition of pink and white gown with a neat cap and badge, all esthetic and antiseptic,"[44] acknowledging nurses as proficient showpieces for a modern hospital hoping to be on the medical cutting edge, but also as models of femininity. Although nursing leaders emphasized education and expertise, the insistence on wearing a uniform as a type of livery put the nurses in a subservient position within the hospital, contributing to what Susan Reverby describes as the failure of nursing to make the transition from "women's sphere to women's rights."[45]

"Rough Diamond into Polished Gem":[46]
Social Class and the Nurse's Uniform

The second, pervading model for the nurses' uniform was the dress of working-class household servants. This model is closely intertwined with that of fashion: nursing borrowed from the vocabulary of fashionable women's dress, but adapted the design and material of the uniform to suit the manual nature of the work and to create a look that was unique to the new occupation.

While the princess-style uniform in figure 7.7 is based on a fashionable style, it is nevertheless associated with the costume worn for women for housecleaning. Instead of being made of delicate cotton or silk, this nurse's dress is made of twill-woven blue denim, first introduced for men's working overalls in the 1850s.[47] A very early example of denim used for women's clothing, this dress is a remarkable combination of fashion and practicality. The choice of fabric for all the schools of nursing established in the late nineteenth century was consistently serviceable, most commonly woven in stripes or printed in patterns of blue and white or pink and white. These colors were made from the two most colorfast dyestuffs available, the blue from indigo and the pink from a synthetic version of madder dye that was available by the late 1870s. These colors would resist fading from frequent washing.

Beyond the practicality of the fiber and color, the fabric for nurses' uniforms proclaimed allegiance to a particular school. Each school went to great lengths to find a fabric that would be unique to that institution. The MGH, for example, began with a pink striped cotton, which they discarded when they found out another Montreal hospital was using the same cloth. They gave up on their second choice of pink-patterned fabric when they found it being worn by an orderly who had purchased the material in Montreal. Finally, they had a specially made fabric imported from England printed with the entwined initials of the hospital.[48] A uniform that is special to its school was one of the most potent ways to inculcate not just loyalty to the school, but also to the hospital. Student nurses really were creatures of their hospitals. The MGH went so far as to "brand" its nurses with the hospital monogram—literally on their bodies.

The princess style of dress was most admired for its ability to emphasize the long slender lines of the female body. This aesthetic ideal was not sustained in the nurse's uniform, due to the voluminous apron tied at the waist, which interrupted the elongation. The apron was the garment that most distinguished nurses from middle-class women of fashion. The "old-time" nurses were, of course, members of the same class as domestic servants, and their hospital tasks were largely those of charwomen. They wore aprons as serviceable garments to protect the fronts of their dresses from soiling. The first Nightingale nurses at St. Thomas's Hospital wore brown holland (unbleached linen) aprons, but most photographs from the 1860s on show nurses wearing white aprons, or some brown and some white. Both brown and white linen or cotton were easily bleached clean, and were frequently changed when dirty.[49]

Photographs of the first nursing schools in North America invariably show snowy white aprons. The white apron has a double message: while it is associated with household work, it is also the color of social contact. It was the custom for household servants to change their rough morning work aprons for the afternoon white starched ones. However, while upper household servants like ladies' maids would wear "a pretty lace-trimmed bib apron," the plain unadorned nursing apron was meant to be hardworking.[50]

By the mid-1890s, most nursing schools in North America added a bib to their aprons. Attached to the apron at the waist, the bib was ostensibly an additional protection for the dress front, but was so stylized as to function more as a sartorial sign of nursing as a new occupation. For example, the WGH uniform included a very stylized narrow bib, with three rows of pleating on either side, and fastened around the neck with a loop (figure 7.12). This and other unique designs for bibs indicate that nursing was beginning to form its own identity.

The first nursing caps were in the style of lady's breakfast or morning caps, worn close to the back of the head, with frilled or goffered edges, and some with streamers down the back. Although women's caps were originally meant to protect the hair from dust, the models for nurses' and maids' caps were decorative rather than practical. But whereas fashionable ladies' caps were made of velvet, lace, and ribbons, the restrained nurses' caps were white, probably made of linen or muslin.[51] Like the princess-style cotton dresses, ladies' caps were meant to be worn in the home. It was unfashionable by the 1870s for middle-class women to wear caps in public. However, caps for nurses, like those for household servants, persisted. As nursing schools proliferated, caps grew in variety and exuberance, the brim changing back and forth from gathered, goffered, and frilled, and the crowns from peaked, triangular, and bifurcated, the fabric from transparent scrim to muslin. These fanciful cap designs for nursing represent another example of a nursing garment that started out as indicating domestic service but became self-referential.

By the 1890s, nurses began to wear detachable collars and cuffs. These practical accessories were introduced in the 1840s and worn exclusively

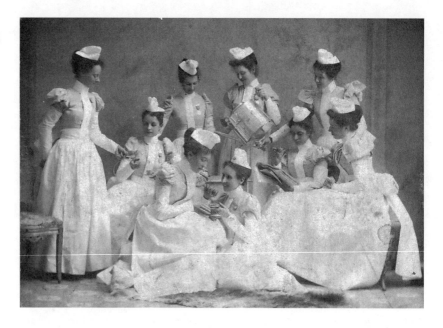

Figure 7.12 Graduating Class, Winnipeg General Hospital School of Nursing, ca. 1895. *Courtesy of the Winnipeg General Hospital and Health Sciences Centre Nurses Alumnae Archives.*

by men, but toward the end of the century, they were appropriated by domestics, typists, and other clerical workers.[52] Nurses were one of the first female occupational groups to adopt a detachable collar and cuffs, likely introduced by nursing superintendents who wished to establish some semblance of a professional image, despite the garments' impracticability. Some of the behind-the-scenes work of cleaning and emptying bedpans was done with cuffs removed and sleeves rolled up, but when on the ward and the in public eye, nurses had to wear the cuffs while giving patients a bath, massage, or liniment rub.[53]

The humble origins of the nurses' uniform were clear, but it also expressed middle-class aspirations. Consider the 1895 photograph of nurses at the WGH (figure 7.12), which describes a group of young women in uniform taking tea. One woman is pouring from a giant teapot, while the rest pass teacups, sip delicately, chat, and read a newspaper. To read this image's conventional or historical meaning, we must be familiar with the cultural codes of the period, through which we can deduce that these uniformed women are student nurses, arranged in a sort of tableau vivant, a popular Victorian parlor game in which guests would pose themselves as works of art or scenes from literary works or history. This was a common motif for group photographs.[54] Their teapot and cups and saucers are props likely brought to the photographer's studio from the nurses' residence.

This tableau can be understood as a performance to persuade the viewer that these student nurses are enacting middle-class ladylike refinement.

Their fresh, clean uniforms and genteel behavior give no hint of the work behind the scenes on the hospital wards. The WGH nurses act as drama-turgical team; as Erving Goffman observes, they were "engaged in main-taining the stability of some definition of the situation, concealing or playing down certain facts."[55] Unlike the old-time nurses, they do not display the tools of their trade, but rather delicate objects divorced from their everyday experiences. The genteel behavior enacted in this photo-graph, divorced from the reality of the work, bypassed another conun-drum in nursing reform: how to explain why the ideal image of the frail and delicate middle-class young woman should take over hospital chores that were the province of hardy and robust matrons?

At the outset, the aim of nursing schools was to attract a "better class of women." Beyond cleanliness and neatness, hospital rules for nurses in-cluded "a quiet manner and becoming demeanour."[56] The need to define nursing as a middle-class, respectable occupation was heightened when hospitals established private wards to attract paying patients by the late 1890s.[57] In order to convince middle-class patients to leave their homes, where they received private nursing care, and enter institutions that were originally intended for the poor, the presence of well-trained and well-behaved nurses whose social status at least appeared to be close to that of the paying patients was crucial. Kathryn McPherson maintains that although the nursing experiment "never achieved the middle-class com-position" that was hoped for, the students were "expected to conform to an elite vision" regardless of their class background.[58]

Nurses' uniforms played a part in this rhetoric. The neatly clothed nurses in figure 7.12—their fashionable silhouettes, perky caps, and per-fectly laundered aprons—reflect a bourgeois sensibility. An often repeated story is told about the uniform at Bellevue nursing school in New York, which, whether true or not, reflects the importance of the uniform as a strategy for class distinctions. From the beginning, Bellevue was an elite school, and in order to establish a dress code, the hospital uniform com-mittee asked a student from an "old and prominent family" to appear in a charming gray-blue striped uniform, white apron, and cap, convincing the rest of the students that their "nondescript print dresses" were "dowdy and insignificant."[59] Good enough for one of Bellevue's posh students, the uniform solved the contradiction of having middle-class women (or women the hospital wanted to appear as middle class) wearing hospital livery like servants.

The appearance of gentility also helped to conceal another nursing reform conundrum: how to make it tolerable for innocent young women to have intimate knowledge of bodies, especially male bodies? This task

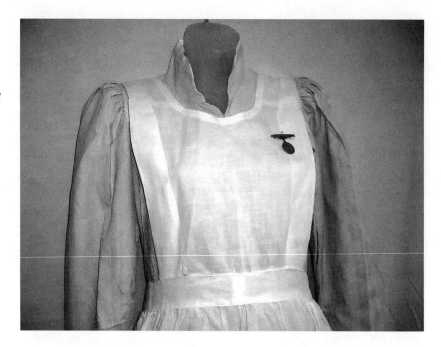

Figure 7.13 Student Uniform, Montreal General Hospital, ca. 1890–1894. *Collection of the Alumnae Association, Montreal General Hospital School of Nursing. Photo © Canadian Museum of Civilization, 2009.122, photo Steven Darby, IMG 2009-0003-0007-Dm.* (Plate 11.)

had been previously accomplished safely by middle-aged matrons who, it was expected, had experience with the carnal. The emphasis on modesty in uniform and behavior that characterized nursing was an attempt to address this problem. Simply wearing a uniform signified that the wearer was required and qualified to do certain tasks that otherwise would be too intrusive for both patient and nurse.

Underneath the veneer of gentility in the WGH tea photograph are the worn and patched uniforms that survive. Figure 7.13 is the bodice of an 1894 MGH uniform made of pink-and-white striped cotton, preserved by the school's alumnae association. It is quite roughly machine sewn, with crude handmade buttonholes. The fabric is very soft and thin from repeated washing, still retaining its pink color, although much faded. There are many tears, especially around the collar, which are roughly darned. This bodice—wash-worn, threadbare, unlined, ripped, and worn until it almost fell apart—is material evidence of the other side of nurses in "pretty pink dresses." It alludes to the need for extreme economy on the part of some of the young students whose families could barely afford to send their daughters to school rather than straight into paying jobs. But even more evocatively, the garment bears witness to the nurse's hard labor of bending, lifting, washing, restraining, and scrubbing.

At the MGH nursing school's inauguration, Dr. Craik assured the hospital's potential sponsors that the hospital had not been extravagant in uniforms for nurses: "That is their working dress. It is not costly; it is not made of silk or satin; indeed, it is made of materials that are quite inexpensive."[60] In the mid-nineteenth century Florence Nightingale stressed the importance of restraint in nursing dress from a practical and moral point of view, but that aim was twisted as reform took hold and clothing the increasing numbers of students became a financial consideration for hospital administrators.

Taking tea was a theme that appears in a remarkable number of nursing photographs. While tableaux like these may have been suggested by the photographer, nurses clearly agreed to their portrayal as genteel ladies. Nursing students may have colluded with nursing reform's construction of class and gender identity, but they were not just passive recipients. Tea-drinking nurses used the hospital's patriarchal system to gain an education and, for women like Isobel Atkinson, to further a career. Moreover, we can imagine that their neat uniforms helped to carve out a place of pride and dignity in a working environment that was exhausting, demanding, and distressing.

Conclusion

Clearly the uniform was fundamental to the modernization of nursing. Every single hospital that established a nurse training school—and most did—immediately adopted a uniform. Nurses in blue or pink uniforms with crisp aprons and puffy caps were paraded in front of community leaders and paying patients. Graduation photographs were proudly hung in the corridor of the nurses' residence to be seen by all the junior students who walked by. The images of nurses played a part in the "'cultural construction' of society ... testimonies of ... social arrangements and above all of ... ways of seeing and thinking."[61]

The nursing uniform's relationship to current fashion was mixed. Nurses were able to signal their youth and sense of style mainly in the sleeve, which ballooned up and down in the 1890s, but fashion was constrained by the serviceable aprons, bibs, and caps. After the first few years, nursing uniforms began to be self-referential. New garments were introduced specifically for nursing, departing from those worn for domestic service or any other trade.

A concrete expression of institutional control, the uniform and the behaviors it required formed a cultural hegemony, which was imposed from above but embraced by students. The uniform was the most potent embodiment of the nurse's identity. The uniform quietly mediated the many challenges faced by nursing reformers. It differentiated and raised the profile of middle-class, or aspiring middle-class, trained nurses who in this early period competed with older working-class practitioners. Representing an occupation that was virtually all female, the uniform retained elements of both domestic service and feminine fashion, thereby reconciling the gender-bending problem of women in the skilled workforce. The uniform disciplined nurses' bodies into appropriate behaviors that would make them efficient and respectable hospital workers.

At the same time as the uniform mediated problems, it held its own contradictions. Was it a symbol of professional status or of subservient submission? Did the demands of "uniformity" restrict or allow young women's self-determination? The first hospital nurse's uniform resists simple interpretation. It was a bricolage based on overlapping models of fashion and servitude. It is a testament to the changing role of women within the vital institution of the hospital as it was transformed by modernization.

Notes

1. Kathryn McPherson, *Bedside Matters: The Transformation of Canadian Nursing*, 1900–1990 (Toronto: Oxford University, 1996), 15.

2. Jennifer Craik, *Uniforms Exposed: From Conformity to Transgression* (London: Berg, 2005), 106.

3. For a discussion of the historiography of the nurse's uniform, and the methodology used in the research for this paper, see Christina Bates, "Looking Closely: Visual and Material Approaches to the Nurse's Uniform," *Nursing History Review* 18 (2008): 167–88.

4. "Mrs. Davis," (obituary) *The Canadian Nurse* 1, no. 4 (Dec 1905), 29, 39, 60 (hereafter cited as "Mrs. Davis," *Canadian Nurse*); Judith Young and Nicole Rousseau, "Lay Nursing from the New France Era to the End of the Nineteenth Century (1608–1891)" (hereafter cited as Young, "Lay Nursing"), in *On All Frontiers: Four Centuries of Canadian Nursing*, ed. Christina Bates, Dianne Dodd, and Nicole Rousseau (Ottawa: University of Ottawa and the Canadian Museum of Civilization, 2005), 24 (hereafter cited as Bates, Dodd, Rousseau, *On All Frontiers*).

5. "Mrs. Davis," *Canadian Nurse*, 29; on early nursing and the Sarah Gamp image, see Katherine Williams, "From Sarah Gamp to Florence Nightingale: A Critical Study of Hospital Nursing Systems from 1840 to 1897," in *Rewriting Nursing History*, ed. Celia Davies (London: Croom Helm, 1980), 41–75; Anne Summers, "The Mysterious Demise of Sarah Gamp: The Domiciliary Nurse and Her Detractors c. 1830–1860," *Victorian Studies* 32, no. 3 (1989), 365–86; Joyce M. MacQueen, "Who the Dickens Brought Sara Gamp to Canada?" *The Canadian Journal of Nursing Research* 21, no. 2 (Summer 1989), 27–36.

6. Carol Helmstadter, "Old Nurses and New: Nursing in the London Teaching Hospitals Before and After the Mid-Nineteenth-Century Reforms," *Nursing History Review* 1 (1993), 43–70; Susan M. Reverby, *Ordered to Care: The Dilemma*

of American Nursing, 1850–1945 (Cambridge: Cambridge University, 1987), 12–36 (hereafter cited as Reverby, *Ordered to Care*); Young, "Lay Nursing."

7. TGH nursing superintendent, Mary Agnes Snively commented that: ". . . most of the nurses were illiterate, and if tradition is to be relied upon, intemperate as well, to say nothing of the impression that prevailed amongst these strong-minded women as a class." Mary Agnes Snively, "The Toronto General Hospital Training School for Nurses," *Canadian Nurse* 1, no. 1 (March, 1905), 7.

8. McGill University Archives, MG 96: Montreal General Hospital School of Nursing Committee of Management Minute Book, July 1, 1889 (hereafter cited as MGH Committee of Management).

9. Glennis Zilm, "Time Line: Kate Miller," work in progress manuscript, July 26, 2006; Glennis Zilm and Sheila Rankin Zerr, "Uniforms Without Uniformity, c. 1874–1895: What the Well-Dressed Canadian Nurse Wore," updated manuscript of presentation given at the 2000 Canadian Association for the History of Nursing Conference, 2006; Sheila J. Rankin Zerr, Glennis Zilm, and Valerie Grant, *Labor of Love: A Memoir of Gertrude Richards Ladner, 1879 to 1976* (Delta, BC: ZGZ Publication, 2006) (hereafter cited as Zerr, Zilm, and Grant, *Labor of Love*).

10. Gordon Dodds, Roger Hall, and Stanley Triggs, *The World of William Notman: The Nineteenth Century Through a Master's Lens* (Boston: David R. Godine, 1992); Peter Hamilton and Roger Hargreaves, eds., *The Beautiful and the Damned: The Creation of Identity in Nineteenth Century Photography* (London: Lund Humphries, 2001). Stanley Triggs, *Portrait of a Period: A Collection of Notman Photographs, 1856–1915* (Montreal: McGill University Press, 1967); and Stanley Triggs, *William Notman: The Stamp of a Studio* (Toronto: Art Gallery of Ontario and Coach House Press, 1985).

11. Ariel Beaujot, "Can Objects Speak? The Glove and the Performance of Middle-Class Womanhood, 1830–1920," (paper presented to the Canadian Historical Association, April 21, 2007), 10, 32–34.

12. Ibid., 20; Michael L. Carlebach, *Working Stiffs: Occupational Portraits in the Age of Tintypes* (Washington: Smithsonian Press, 2002).

13. *Training School for Nurses in Connection with the Montreal General Hospital, Formal Opening* (Montreal: Gazette Printing Company, 1890), 5 (hereafter cited as MGH Formal Opening).

14. On the introduction of the first training schools, see Kathryn McPherson, "The Nightingale Influence and the Rise of the Modern Hospital" (hereafter cited as McPherson, "Nightingale Influence"); and Lynn Kirkwood, "Enough but Not Too Much: Nursing Education in English Language Canada (1874–2000)," in Bates, Dodd, Rousseau, *On All Frontiers*, 73–87 and 183–95.

15. Nathan Joseph, *Uniforms and Nonuniforms: Communication Through Clothing* (New York: Greenwood, 1986), 14.

16. Poplin, Irene Schuessler, "Nursing Uniforms: Romantic Idea, Functional Attire, or Instrument of Social Change?" *Nursing History Review* 2 (1994), 153–67.

17. Elizabeth Ewing, *Women in Uniform Through the Centuries* (London: B.T. Batsford, 1975), 37–38 (hereafter cited as Ewing, *Women in Uniform*); Sarah A. Tooley, *The History of Nursing in the British Empire* (London: S.H. Bousfield, 1906), 36, 62.

18. Ewing, *Women in Uniform*, 44.

19. Gayle V. Fischer, *Pantaloons and Power: A Nineteenth-Century Dress Reform in the United States* (Kent, Ohio: Kent State University, 2001), 24.

20. Patricia A. Cunningham, *Reforming Women's Fashion, 1850–1920: Politics, Health, and Art* (Kent, Ohio: Kent State University, 2003), 1 (hereafter cited as Cunningham, *Reforming Women*).

21. *History of Mack Training School for Nurses, Seventy-Fifth Anniversary, 1874–1949* (St. Catharines: The Alumnae Association, 1949), 21–22; Margaret Isabel Lawrence, *History of the School for Nurses, Toronto General Hospital* (Toronto: The Alumnae Association, [1931]), 10 (hereafter cited as Lawrence, *TGH History*).

22. See, for example, "Ladies' Walking and Evening Dresses," Stella Blum, ed., *Victorian Fashions and Costumes from Harper's Bazaar, 1867–1898* (New York, Dover, 1974), 163 (hereafter cited as Blum, *Harper's Bazaar*).

23. Lawrence, *TGH History*, 10.

24. Florence Nightingale, *Notes on Hospitals* (London: Longman, Green, Longman, Roberts, and Green, 1863), 8–11; Charles E. Rosenberg, "Florence Nightingale on Contagion: The Hospital as Moral Universe," in *Explaining Epidemics and Other Studies in the History of Medicine*, ed. Charles E. Rosenberg (Cambridge: Cambridge University Press, 1992); Michael Worboys, *Spreading Germs: Disease Theories and Medical Practice in Britain, 1865–1900* (Cambridge: Cambridge University Press, 2000).

25. Florence Nightingale, *Notes on Nursing: What It Is, and What It is Not* (New York: Appleton, 1860), 127.

26. Ewing, *Women in Uniform*, 43.

27. Jane Brooks and Anne Marie Rafferty, "Dress and Distinction in Nursing, 1860–1939: 'A Corporate (as well as corporeal) Armour of Probity and Purity,'" *Women's History Review* 16, no.1 (February 2007): 41–57.

28. See, for example, Valerie Steele, *The Corset: A Cultural History* (New Haven: Yale University Press, 2001); Leigh Summers, *Bound to Please: A History of the Victorian Corset* (Oxford: Berg, 2001).

29. *Nursing Record*, December 13, 1888, 536.

30. Cunningham, *Reforming Women*, 147–48.

31. John Berger, *Ways of Seeing*, 1972, quoted in Gillian Rose, *Visual Methodologies: An Introduction to the Interpretation of Visual Materials* (London: Sage, 2001), 24; see also Peter Burke, *Eyewitnessing: The Uses of Images as Historical Evidence* (Ithaca, NY: Cornell University, 2001), 179 (hereafter cited as Burke, *Eyewitnessing*).

32. Dan W. Blumhagen, "The Doctor's White Coat: The Image of the Physician in Modern America," *Annals of Internal Medicine* 91 (1979), 111–16; MGH Committee of Management, May 11, 1891; January 31, 1896.

33. Kathryn McPherson, "The Case of the Kissing Nurse: Sexuality and Sociability in Canadian Nursing, 1920–1967," in *Gendered Pasts: Historical Essays on Femininity and Masculinity in Canada*, ed. Kathryn McPherson, Cecilia Morgan and Nancy Forestell (Toronto: Oxford University, 1999), 183.

34. H. E. MacDermot, *History of the School of Nursing of the Montreal General Hospital* (Montreal: The Alumnae Association, 1940), 49 (hereafter cited as Mac-Dermot, *MGH History*).

35. Ibid., 110; MGH Committee of Management, September 7 and 14, 1891.

36. Jane Hodson, *How to be a Trained Nurse: A Manual of Information in Detail* (New York: W. Abbatt, 1898), 85.

37. Quoted in Margaret M. Street, *Watch-fires on the Mountains: The Life and Writings of Ethel Johns* (Toronto: University of Toronto, 1973), 23.

38. MacDermot, *MGH History*, 118.

39. Anne Pearson, *The Royal Jubilee Hospital School of Nursing, 1891–1982* (Victoria, BC: Alumnae Association, 1985), 8.

40. MGH Formal Opening, 10–11.

41. Pauline O. Jardine, "An Urban Middle-Class Calling: Women and the Emergence of Modern Nursing Education at the Toronto General Hospital, 1881–1914," *Urban History Review*, 17, no. 3 (February 1989): 176–190. (hereafter cited as Jardine, "An Urban Middle-Class Calling").

42. MGH Formal Opening, 8.

43. McPherson, "The Nightingale Influence," 78–79.

44. McGill University Archives, MG 96: Montreal General Hospital, Minutes of the Board of Governors, 1890, quoted in H. E. MacDermot, MGH History, 43.

45. Reverby, *Ordered to Care*, 58.

46. "Nurses' Life in the Montreal General Hospital," *Dominion Illustrated Monthly Magazine* 1, no. 9 (October 1892), 543.

47. Webster's dictionary of 1864 referred to denim as "a coarse cotton drilling used for overalls, etc."; Lynn Downey, "A Short History of Denim," http://www.levistrauss.com/Downloads/History-Denim.pdf.

48. MacDermot, *MGH History*, 43.

49. Ewing, *Women in Uniform*, 46.

50. Phyllis Cunnington and Catherine Lucas, *Occupational Costume in England* (London: Adam and Charles Black, 1976), 213.

51. See, for example, "Caps" in Blum, *Harper's Bazaar*, 33.

52. Michael J. Murphy, "Orthopedic Manhood: Detachable Shirt Collars and the Reconstruction of the White Male Body in America, ca. 1880–1910," *Dress* 32 (2005), 75–95.

53. Alice Dannatt, "Clothing for the Nursing Staff of a Hospital," *Nursing Record* (November 22, 1888), 476.

54. Cynthia Cooper, *Magnificent Entertainments: Fancy Dress Balls of Canada's Governors General, 1876–1896* (Fredericton, NB: Goose Lane Editions and the Canadian Museum of Civilization, 1997), 22, 41, 69; Heinz K. Henisch and Brigit A. Henisch, *The Photographic Experience, 1839–1914: Images and Attitudes* (Philadelphia: Pennsylvania State University Press, 1994), 70–71, 354.

55. Erving Goffman, *The Presentation of Self in Everyday Life* (Garden City, NY: Doubleday Anchor, 1959), 105.

56. Zerr, Zilm, and Grant, *Labor of Love*, 53.

57. Jardine, "An Urban Middle-Class Calling," 182.

58. McPherson, *Bedside Matters*, 17–18.

59. M. Adelaine Nutting and Lavinia L. Dock, *A History of Nursing*, vol. 2 (New York: G.P. Putnam's Sons, 1907–1912), 401.

60. MGH Formal Opening, 29.

61. Burke, *Eyewitnessing*, 185.

❧ 8

THE FACE OF FASHION

Race and Fantasy in James VanDerZee's Photography
and Jessie Fauset's Fiction

In 1926, W. E. B. Du Bois asked leading publishers, artists, and intellectuals, most of whom were associated with what came to be known as the Harlem Renaissance, to write responses to the question "The Negro in Art: How Shall He Be Portrayed?" The resulting essays were published in the NAACP's *Crisis* magazine, of which Du Bois was the editor-in-chief. Du Bois contributed a concluding essay, "Criteria of Negro Art," which famously asserted, "all art is propaganda" and called on artists to create depictions of African-Americans that countered prevailing racist stereotypes.[1] As Du Bois's question and answer suggest, the issue of portraiture and its form became a matter of pressing political import in a period in which artists and intellectuals sought to alter the image of African-Americans and thus "reconstruct the very *idea* of who or what a Negro was or could be."[2] Given the legacy of depicting African-Americans through caricature, mimicry, or racialist science, making an African-American the subject of a dignified artistic portrait could be perceived as a form of aesthetic and political intervention.[3]

Among the influential figures Du Bois approached to write these editorials were activist and philanthropist Joel Spingarn, publisher Alfred Knopf, Sr., cultural critic H. L. Mencken, writer Charles Chesnutt, and the *Crisis*'s literary editor, Jessie Fauset, who was one of the only women asked to contribute. Indeed, the debate was framed in largely masculine terms. Yet, as recent scholarship on the Harlem Renaissance has demonstrated, competing ideas about how one could and should portray African-American women also shaped the visual, literary, and musical culture of the period, from the fiction of Nella Larsen to the music of Mamie Smith.[4] Cherene Sherrard-Johnson, for example, has recently explored how African-American painters in the 1920s and 1930s, such as Archibald J. Motley, Jr., addressed questions of racial identity, inheritance, and female sexuality through their portraits of the "New Negro Woman."[5] Moreover, while artists were experimenting with modes of representation, the ways that "ordinary" women performed particular ideas of femininity and race were treated as a matter of collective concern. Church and intellectual leaders critiqued certain fashions and beauty practices while, in the *Crisis*, editorials about how the "Negro" should be portrayed ran alongside images of neatly dressed African-American women, which implicitly signaled how the "New Negro woman" should "portray" herself through her clothing and beauty practices.[6]

Feminist critics have long noted that modernity is marked by women's spectacularization and objectification.[7] In the case of African-American women in the early twentieth century, these associations amongst femininity, visuality, and materiality intersected with debates about the political import of representing the self and the race. Thus, black women faced a particular burden of appearing—that is, of deploying their own status as spectacular objects and as types or representatives of a collectivity. In this chapter, I examine this gendered labor of self-fashioning as it is explored in the photography of James VanDerZee and the fiction of Jessie Fauset. I propose that VanDerZee and Fauset's work uses fashion to examine the interplay of subject and object, individual and collective, which, they suggest, is central to African-American women's experience of modernity. In turn, through their treatments of fashion, VanDerZee and Fauset imagine what forms of agency, individuality, and transformation are possible (and, to them, desirable) within these cultural conditions.

Explorations of fashion and of photography during the Harlem Renaissance have only begun to be integrated into analyses of the broader cultural and political trends of the period.[8] Both VanDerZee and Fauset also remain peripheral to scholarship on the Harlem Renaissance, in part because of the perceived stylistic and cultural conservatism of their work; both artists draw on "Victorian" aesthetic practices, and they emphasize respectability, propriety, and prosperity in many of their works. These aesthetic values have proved more difficult to integrate into the narrative of experimentation and iconoclasm that shapes accounts of Harlem in the Jazz Age.[9] Fauset's work, in particular, has been described as ideologically and aesthetically stifled, though such views are beginning to be complicated by recent scholars.[10] This relative critical neglect notwithstanding, both artists had exceptionally prolific careers and played significant (though quite different) roles in the cultural life of Harlem. The first black female graduate of Cornell, Fauset served as literary editor of the *Crisis* from 1919 to 1926. In that period, the magazine published work by most of the influential writers associated with the Renaissance, and Fauset was an important advocate and mentor for many of these artists, including Langston Hughes. She produced four novels and numerous short stories, which draw upon conventions of popular romance. Many of her works—including "The Sleeper Wakes" (1920), *There is Confusion* (1924), *Plum Bun* (1929), and *The Chinaberry Tree* (1931)—feature black women who make their living through dress and fashion. Fashion is also central to the work of VanDerZee, a largely self-taught photographer who operated a studio in Harlem from 1916 to 1969. He catered to walk-in clients and took on commissioned work, including acting as the official photographer for Marcus Garvey's United Negro Improvement Association (UNIA) in the mid-1920s.[11] Residents and visitors to Harlem came to VanDerZee's studio in order to create images of themselves as individuals and as part of the imagined urban community of Harlem, a space that had come to symbolize the hope for African-Americans' improving economic and social conditions in the early twentieth century. VanDerZee draws upon traditions of nineteenth-century portraiture, and in his photographs, such as *Three Generations* (1934), dress emerges as a primary means for the subjects of these photographs to imagine and present themselves as notable individuals, as members of a race, and as denizens of Harlem (figure 8.3).

Indeed, fashion and studio photography offer particularly rich mediums for reading the interplay of individual and collective, which is central to the construction of racial identity and to attempts to alter the portrayal of African-Americans in this period.[12] As the introduction to this volume notes, Georg Simmel claimed that fashion expressed and reconciled the competing impulses toward singularity and conformity that characterize life in a modern democracy.[13] Simmel's analysis helps to illuminate why VanDerZee and Fauset draw on fashion as they attempt to reconcile the pursuit of personal pleasure, an ideology of individual accomplishment as well as an embrace of fantasies of self-transformation, with a regard for women's duties to their imagined racial community. Like fashion, studio portrait photography is at once an object for private consumption and public display, a form of art and a commercial medium. It, too, is a highly conventional mode of generating an image of the self and is a means both of individualization and conformity.

According to Roland Barthes, the tension between specificity and abstraction is intrinsic to photography as a whole. Barthes suggests that "a photograph cannot signify (aim at a generality) except by assuming a mask," that is, an abstract concept or type (unless we are acquainted with the referent or subject of the photograph).[14] VanDerZee's photographs

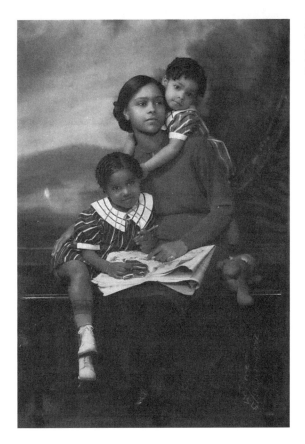

Figure 8.1 James VanDerZee (1886–1983). [untitled], 1936. *Courtesy of Donna Mussenden VanDerZee.*

dramatize this process of transforming specific subjects into "types" through their composition, as his studio space and props transform his sitters into the protagonists of recognizable bourgeois domestic scenes. VanDerZee sometimes sold his studio photographs to companies compiling photographic calendars, and his images often attempt to create a narrative through props and poses.[15] In a photograph dated 1936, for example, an attractive, well-dressed woman poses over a newspaper with two children, so as to suggest that they are in the midst of a cozy domestic scene (figure 8.1). The children are dressed in matching outfits, which complement their mother's stylish dress, and it appears that VanDerZee has also etched in identical bracelets around the children's wrists, which adds to the air of prosperity and order. The composition of the image and its pleasing symmetry combine to make this woman an icon of youthful maternity. Such photographs appear to divorce subjects from the material conditions of their "real" lives and to conceal the individual's "actual" class position. Yet, in doing so, these techniques actually highlight the inextricability of the subject from its material conditions, for they rely on objects to make and remake the self.

In her work, 9 Props (1995), contemporary artist Lorna Simpson comments upon VanDerZee's use of objects in his photography (figure 8.2). In this piece, Simpson has reproduced nine photographs on felt with captions below each image, which give the title and a brief description of a photograph by VanDerZee. The photographs are not VanDerZee's, however; rather, Simpson has chosen a single object (such as a vase or bowl) from a photograph by VanDerZee, had it reproduced in black glass, and then photographed it against a simple, light background. While these explicit references to VanDerZee help to recover and acknowledge the legacy of his work, 9 Props offers a critique of the ways that VanDerZee's subjects (particularly his female subjects) operate as "props" in the construction of particular images of African-American life.[16] By replacing subjects with objects, Simpson draws attention to the ways that the accoutrements of bourgeois life (such as vases and glasses) come to overwhelm the people in VanDerZee's photographs.

Yet 9 Props also prompts us to perceive the dynamic and interdependent relationships between subject and object that emerge in VanDerZee's images, such as the untitled image of the woman with her children and Three Generations. In this photograph, as in many of VanDerZee's works, any opposition between props and human subjects is complicated by the emphasis on clothing to generate a narrative about the figures in the image. As an intimate object usually selected and likely fashioned to some extent by the sitters themselves, clothing highlights the subject's participation in constructing the prosthetic apparatus of subjectivity even in the context of VanDerZee's highly directorial technique.[17] Attention to clothing in VanDerZee's photographs thus intersects with recent critical attention to "things" and with a substantial body of feminist theory, which interrogate the concept of the autonomous modern subject by tracing the interdependence of subject and object.[18] VanDerZee's images, as well as Fauset's fiction, emphasize the inseparability of the gendered and raced subject and its material—and specifically sartorial—conditions. In this way, African-American women and their relationship to clothing become paradigmatic of VanDerZee's vision of modern life.

In VanDerZee and Fauset's work, the subject's dependence on material objects is not solely a condition of compulsion and constraint. Both artists attempt to imagine how clothing in particular admits possibilities for adjusting the norms and practices of race and gender and even for play and pleasure. Accordingly, while neither artist mounts a radical critique of the norms and practices of race and gender in modernity, they treat these categories skeptically and they imagine, through their use of romance and fantasy, new configurations and new possibilities within the sphere

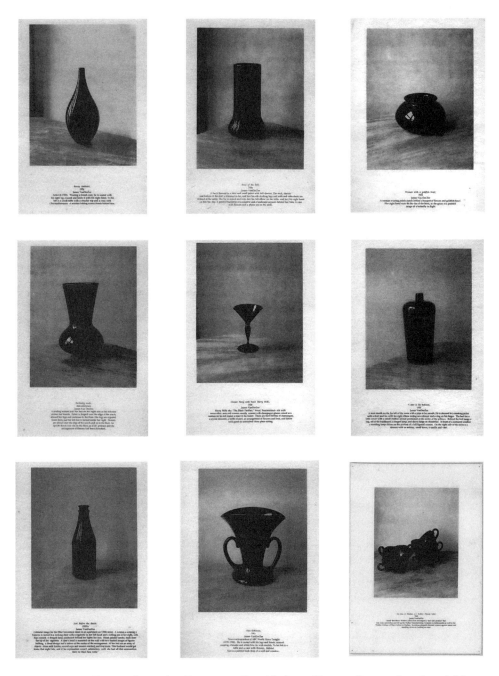

Figure 8.2 Lorna Simpson (b. 1960). *9 Props*, 1995. *Copyright Lorna Simpson. Courtesy the artist and Salon94.*

of the everyday. Moreover, as VanDerZee's images register and respond to his sitter's self-fashioning through clothing, and as Fauset depicts female characters with a passionate interest in dress, their work validates women's labor in portraying the self and "the race" as part of a vision of racial progress. These tactics of negotiation, legitimation, and adaptation are reflected in their use of seemingly conventional aesthetic forms to depict African-Americans, who were decidedly unconventional subjects for dignified photographic and literary portraiture. In addition, their work shows that changing dress was pivotal to efforts to establish African-Americans as subjects of portraits, rather than cartoons, ethnography, or minstrelsy.[19]

Fashioning the African-American Family

Critics have described VanDerZee and Fauset's work as more "Victorian" or "Edwardian" than modern, in part because of their romantic style.[20] Scholars note that VanDerZee's props and backdrops as well as his sitter's poses drew from techniques of late nineteenth-century portrait photography (such as pictorialism), as well as commercial portrait photography (VanDerZee began his career as a studio photographer at a department store).[21] His technique of hiding physical "flaws" by retouching images to bring out what he termed his sitters' "best selves" has prompted readings of his work as a rather prim or narrow expression of the ideology of racial uplift (which emerged in the nineteenth century), though such views have become less prevalent as recent critics have come to explore the artistic and experimental aspects of his work.[22] VanDerZee and Fauset's interest in fashion has been linked to their use of late nineteenth-century aesthetic practices. Kobena Mercer, for example, notes that Van-DerZee "retained the full-length figure of the turn of the century, which widened his range of compositional choices for the 'staging' of his subjects. This approach gave VanDerZee a broader canvas on which to exercise his understanding of the language of clothes."[23] Fauset's detailing of dress and fashion appear to follow the conventions of romance developed in the nineteenth century and continued in "middlebrow" fiction of the early twentieth century. She employs elements of romantic and sentimental genres to explore the lives and loves of African-American men and women, and her stories appear to endorse moral values—such as industriousness, feminine chastity, and women's modesty—which are associated with the American middle class. This view is exemplified by Langston Hughes's description of Fauset in his autobiography *The Big Sea* as one of the people who "midwived the so-called New Negro literature into being" by nurturing younger writers while she served as the literary editor of the *Crisis*.[24] Hughes's verb suggests something of why Fauset has received less attention than, for example, Zora Neale Hurston and Nella Larsen. In contrast to Hurston's bold treatment of female sexuality and to Larsen's modernist narrative style, Fauset's work can appear antiquated, snugly domestic, and apolitical. Following the work of Deborah E. Mc-Dowell and others, however, recent scholars have shown the ways in which Fauset's seemingly simple narratives critique constraints on women's sexuality and desire, challenge racial binaries, and explore the limits of citizenship and racial uplift.[25] My chapter builds on this scholarship by showing how Fauset's work casts a critical eye on women's ability to accept, defy, and remake the burden of "representing" the race, particularly through the production and consumption of fashion. VanDerZee and Fauset's engagement with dress and portraiture emphasizes a paradox of racial distinctions—that while they depend upon fantasy, they are also maintained through often invisible material labor and they render very palpable effects.

Part of the seeming conservatism of VanDerZee and Fauset's work is the apparent idealization of bourgeois family values. In their concern with reproduction, inheritance, and their portraits of African-American families, their art registers and responds to popular discourses about eugenics and racial progress, which scholars have recently explored in more canonical and experimental texts associated with the Harlem Renaissance and modernism.[26] Yet VanDerZee and Fauset's focus on dress's role in the establishment and perpetuation of generational ties and a particular vision of the family also works to expose the tenuousness and vulnerability of the bonds of inheritance and blood. As a potentially shifting signifier of identity, fashion at once expresses and undermines the class, race, and gender distinctions that eugenic theories held were not changeable but, rather, natural and immutable.

The fashioning of the family emerges in VanDerZee's *Three Generations*, which shows five women of various ages carefully posed and dressed for what appears to be a family portrait (figure 8.3). This focus on generational progression is a recurring theme in VanDerZee's work, as for example when he used photomontage to suggest the ghostly presence of past or future generations. This photograph, however, is unusual in that it captures the presence of three generations and focuses solely on women. The image's matrilineal narrative is reinforced through the composition of the figures, which helps to emphasize similarities among the women's facial features as well as their dress. Indeed, the women's clothing and positioning tells a story of familial relationships, as there is a family resemblance among the wide, triangular collars of four of the women's

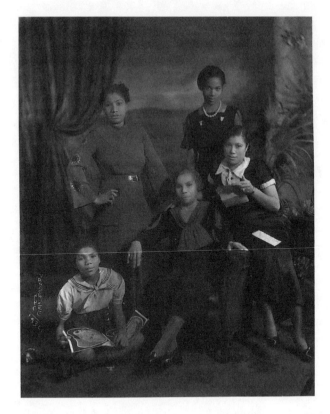

outfits; the women's harmonious outfits and similar sense of style suggests shared values and sensibilities. The family "line of descent" is represented by the young girl's position below and below the women, and her
white blouse picks up on and amplifies the collar of the woman on the
other side of the group. Dress thus articulates and consolidates the relationship between these women and announces the capacity of the African-American family to reconstruct and maintain itself through these
material bonds. At the same time, the use of dress to reinforce these connections speaks to the vulnerability of the narratives of inheritance and
racial identity upon which the African-American family rests at this
time.[27] In this sense, VanDerZee's photograph reveals a tension between
"face" and "frock"—between purportedly stable racial signifiers and fashionable visual cues that are characterized by their mutability and modernity. The prominence of and attention to dress in VanDerZee's images
underscores the malleable and fantastic nature of modern racial and gender identity and its reliance on external cues and props. In VanDerZee's
work, fashion's connection to artifice and femininity enables it, paradoxically, to illuminate the work of fantasy that underpins racial identity.

Fauset also considers how dress symbolizes and maintains familial connections among African-American women and constructs fantasies of African-American femininity. A number of her stories and novels—including "The Sleeper Wakes" (1920), *Plum Bun*, and *The Chinaberry Tree*—feature female characters with an "innate" and extraordinary taste in clothing. In the novels, Fauset shows that this eye for fashion is shared with other female relatives and forms a bond amongst sisters, mothers, and daughters. Fauset shows that this skill is not merely frivolous, but allows the women to support themselves (and, in the case of *The Chinaberry Tree*, their families as well). This is not to say that Fauset simply celebrates fashion as a source of familial connection and financial support. Critics who have discussed Fauset's sustained interest in women's dress and feminine beauty often describe her as hostile to its seductions and solipsism. For example, in a recent essay entitled "Beauty Along the Color Line," Russ Castronovo contrasts Du Bois's conviction that beauty can accomplish political aims with what he asserts is Fauset's dismissal of its power. As evidence, Castronovo cites a scene in "The Sleeper Wakes" in which the protagonist, a very fair woman who belatedly discovers that she is probably African-American, finds that her physical beauty cannot persuade her white husband not to attack a black male servant. Castronovo concludes that though Fauset is "usually a staunch ally of Du Bois," here she demonstrates that "[s]tigmatized as feminine, beauty has no role to play in the defense of black masculinity."[28] However, Castronovo's contrast occludes her nuanced view of the political significance of women's beauty and appearance. In "The Sleeper Wakes," for example, Fauset actually offers a more qualified understanding of how the manipulation and deployment of feminine beauty can aid not men but women. After her husband divorces her when she tells him she is probably African-American, the heroine's innate sense of sartorial beauty and style enables her to get a job at a couture house, which serves a wealthy white clientele. There the heroine demonstrates that she has an extraordinary mastery of the sartorial codes of the modern elite. Many working-class African-American women supported themselves by "taking in" sewing or working as seamstresses, and in this tale, Fauset refigures this legacy of need and compulsion into an inherited skill that opens up possibilities for her heroine and demonstrates her mastery of the sartorial codes that shape modern high society. This talent helps to reconnect her with her racial identity and offers a key source of support—though, significantly, not liberation or lasting independence. The heroine chooses to leave her job at the fashion house so that she can reunite with the African-American family that had adopted and raised her from a young age. In "The Sleeper Wakes," the display of women's beauty may be useless or ineffectual, but the production of beauty grants African-American women a means of economic power and signals their facility with the sartorial codes of the modern.

Aesthetics and Imitation

The appearance in Fauset's novels of so many female characters who work as dressmakers, designers, and (in one case) a fashion illustrator for white clients raises the question of imitation—that is, whether an interest in fashion amounts to a desire to mimic "white" cultural values. Moreover, because VanDerZee and Fauset employ older and relatively conservative aesthetic forms, they can be read as adopting ideals associated with the white middle-class.[29] Indeed, anxieties about imitation emerged in both the artistic and beauty culture of the Harlem Renaissance. Adopting the language of dress in "Criteria of Negro Art," for example, Du Bois balanced his call for dignified representations of African-Americans with a warning that artists and readers should not adopt "customs that have come down as second-hand soul clothes of white patrons," such as a prudish shame at the mention of sex, or excessive piety.[30] Meanwhile, interest in fashion on the part of African-American women was often critiqued as a desire to copy "white" lifestyles.[31] These readings inflect later examinations of VanDerZee and Fauset's work. Perhaps most egregiously, Barthes claims that VanDerZee's *Family Portrait* (1926) "utters respectability, family life, conformism, Sunday best, an effort of social advancement in order to assume the White Man's attributes."[32]

Fauset's novels *Plum Bun* and *The Chinaberry Tree*, as well as VanDerZee's *Three Generations*, confront the issue of imitation explicitly and attempt to challenge the primacy of dominant conceptions of beauty and style in part by focusing on African-American women's mastery of sartorial codes. They trouble readings of artists, intellectuals, and ordinary individuals' investment in consumer culture and fashion during the Harlem Renaissance as an effort to conform to "white" styles and mores.[33] Fauset, VanDerZee, and his subjects construct a sartorial and artistic aesthetic, which draws from disparate traditions to recast prevailing (and implicitly white) forms of photography, fiction, and femininity. As critics have begun to explore, VanDerZee and Fauset did not simply imitate older forms or promulgate ideas of racial uplift, but instead adopted and remade traditional modes of narrative and portraiture. They combined older elements with more modern details, and this amalgamation between tradition and modernity is often dramatized through their depictions of dress.

The heroine of *The Chinaberry Tree*, for example, unites a cutting-edge taste in fashion with a firmly conventional sense of sexual and social propriety. This contrast between fashionability and traditionalism plays out not only in Laurentine's character, but also in the contrast between Laurentine's very modern dress (which she designs) and her staid, prosperous hometown with its well-heeled black inhabitants. The juxtaposition plays out as in a VanDerZee studio portrait; the stuffy Victorian mores of the town set off Laurentine's modernity while situating her in a realm of cozy middle-class life. Laurentine's skill as a fashion designer also serves as a way for Fauset to complicate the alignment of fashion with whiteness. Focusing not only on the consumption but also on the production of fashion, Fauset depicts black women as creating the styles and modes that they also follow. Laurentine possesses an innate and exquisite taste, which helps her to develop a successful business creating clothing for upper middle-class white women from rich New Jersey towns. The novel emphasizes that the white suburban women not only buy Laurentine's designs, but also rely on her fashion sense so that Laurentine becomes a trusted expert on what is modern, fashionable, and appropriate. While establishing the influence exerted by Laurentine's fashion sense, Fauset's novel also insists on a connection between style and character and suggests that dress plays a pivotal role in the way that women negotiate their own class, racial, and gender position within modernity. Fauset's treatment thus contests the ideas of fashion as imitation, blind conformity, or irrationality and discovers a modest role of authority for African-American women. Susan Tomlinson has aligned Laurentine's sale of her designs to white clients with Fauset's attempt in *Plum Bun* to package a vision of middle-class black life, which will appeal to white consumers of the novel. Tomlinson observes, moreover, that Laurentine finds a strong community once she begins to design for the bourgeois black women who befriend her. Fauset's narrative itself, Tomlinson proposes, may have appealed to black audiences in part as a kind of "conduct manual," which forged a sense of community around this black aesthetic that bears the approval of white publishers and audiences.[34] Tomlinson cautions that Fauset must not have been explicitly promoting "[s]uch a didactic, embarrassingly Booker-T.-Washingtonian, 'topsheets and toothbrushes' approach to uplift."[35] But by building on her reading we can see that Laurentine's fashion sense does, on some level, do the work that Du Bois envisioned for art in "Criteria of Negro Art," in that it helps to present or fashion African-

Americans in a way that counters racist iconography. Tomlinson's reading thus helps us to realize that Fauset's vision recuperates fashion as a means of forging community and shared cultures of femininity. In doing so, Fauset contests the alignment of fashion with narcissism and individual desire, an association which Du Bois makes in "Criteria of Negro Art" when he contrasts a petty greed for "the most striking clothes" and "the richest dinners" with what he claims is African-Americans' true craving for beauty and culture.[36]

In making Laurentine a fashion designer, Fauset imagines for her an agency and artistry that goes beyond her roles as a symbol or projection of a racial ideal—or an imitation of whiteness. At the same time, by creating a sense of community and pride around Laurentine's creations, *The Chinaberry Tree* helps to legitimate the political work performed by the production and consumption of fashion. Moreover, Fauset's emphasis on the pleasure that Laurentine's creations give her and her black clients implicitly challenges the assumption that such personal delights are antithetical to an appreciation of true beauty and to the aims of racial uplift. Fauset draws upon fashion to reconcile pleasure and duty in her vision of the lives of middle-class black women.

In *Three Generations*, an image of fashionable white femininity has been inserted into this family portrait. As in many VanDerZee images, the sleek, modern (if conservative) dress of the subjects contrasts with the old-fashioned setting of the studio with its painted backdrop of a landscape, heavy drapes, and fern; the background and VanDerZee's arrangement of the women helps to set their modern self-fashioning in relief. VanDerZee has structured the image around the carefully tailored dress of one woman, who displays almost the full length of her elegant outfit and places a hand on her hip so as to show off the unusual design on her sleeve. This demonstration of fashionability appears as a form of confident self-assertion. At the same time, the photograph contains a seemingly very different model of fashionable femininity. VanDerZee has staged the scene so that the young girl seems to be looking up from perusing illustrations of white women with stylish haircuts. This arrangement invites a comparison between the printed illustrations and the forms of femininity and fashion enacted by the girl's own family members. VanDerZee's image offers a response to the supposed superiority of these white models of beauty by emphasizing the pride and the familial and cultural ties among these women. At the same time, by producing this picture of this family, VanDerZee participates in the reproduction and circulation of alternative forms of feminine beauty. The presence of the letter in the hand of one of the sisters underscores this sense of the circulation of cultural ideas and values, as it signals her participation in a wider community of letters, ideas, and perhaps professional accomplishments. The women demonstrate their mastery of sartorial and social codes, as well as their confidence in their own performance of fashionable femininity. Thus, even as VanDerZee's photograph reminds the viewer of the association between fashionability and whiteness, his image invites us to recognize the achievement and challenges of these women as they follow, defy, and remake prevailing sartorial and social values and situate themselves in a generational history of African-American women.

Reconciling Pleasure and Racial Politics

While in *The Chinaberry Tree* Fauset redeems fashion from its apparent solipsism and apoliticism, *Plum Bun* more directly observes the distinctions between art and fashion, personal pleasure and racial politics. The novel examines whether an appreciation for stylish dress should be understood as an "aesthetic sense" akin to an appreciation for art, and it appears to chart a progression away from fashion toward high art and racial consciousness. Yet the novel's romantic and improbable conclusion stages a fantastic reconciliation among art, activism, and accoutrement, and in doing so it refuses to relinquish the pleasures of fashion in ways that resonate with VanDerZee's use of glamour and fantasy, such as in the photograph *Before the Night Out* (1930), which I discuss below. *Plum Bun* fuses a passing narrative and a popular romance with an artist's coming-of-age story. The heroine, Angela Murray, leaves her darker-skinned sister to move to New York, where she passes as white in order to pursue her ambitions as an artist. She supports herself as a fashion illustrator while taking painting classes. In *Plum Bun*, Angela's career as a fashion illustrator is clearly distinguished from her burgeoning career as a portrait artist and her growing racial consciousness, which is spurred by the injustices suffered by a fellow African-American art student. Indeed her job as an illustrator abruptly ends when she reveals her racial background and is fired. The novel is at pains to establish that her interest in the fashionable life of white society emerges from her brief childhood experiences of passing on shopping excursions with her light-skinned mother. Thus, although Angela's capabilities as a fashion illustrator rely on the same inherited "eye for line" and "feeling for colour" that her portraits express, they are clearly an inferior use of her natural talents, just as her innate beauty is misused as a ticket or "pass" into fashionable white society.[37]

Angela's abilities as a portrait artist, on the other hand, lend themselves to the sort of reparative, propagandistic work that Du Bois describes in

"Criteria of Negro Art." Angela's talent is for painting "types" and "writ[ing] down a history with her brush" (112). Her rather traditional realist style expresses the sense of "Truth and Justice" that Du Bois's "Criteria" claimed was essential to art as it documents social conditions through nuanced, penetrating, and sympathetic images of individuals.[38] Her portraits not only capture the superficial markers of race and countenance but also interpret "the emotion which lay back of that expression" (111). Accordingly, Angela's understanding of her subjects develops with her own suffering, and after years of study and personal disappointment she wins the scholarship to study painting at Fontainebleau for her painting of "Fourteenth Street Types," which emerges from her sympathy and growing identification with the immigrants and "shabby pedestrians" she encounters in Greenwich Village.

As Fauset's treatment of Angela underscores, strategies of representation took on political meaning, as formal experimentation was perceived to be in tension, at times, with the aims of presenting particular images of African-Americans. In Du Bois's "Criteria" and in the aesthetic experiments of *Fire!!* magazine, for example, an avant-garde rejection of traditional narrative forms was seen as a refusal to bring representational strategies in line with attempts to gain political representation for African-Americans.[39] Fauset's description of Angela's realist style clearly validates the use of traditional modes of portraying individuals as a means of progressive political intervention. As scholars have noted, the title of Angela's award-winning work clearly aligns her with the Fourteenth Street School of painters, who created realist images of working-class inhabitants of urban New York (often women) going about their daily lives.[40] Yet Fauset's emphasis on her art as a way of recording "history" and registering "types" also echoes discourses about the nature and purposes of photography in this period. Since the publication of Jacob Riis's *How the Other Half Lives: Studies Among the Tenements of New York* (1890), photography was widely recognized as an exemplary medium for exposing the "truth" of urban existence that fell beyond the purview of the white middle class. Emphasizing photography's documentary function, Walter Benjamin further claimed that photography could help individuals to grapple with the anonymity and mutability of urban life by helping them to perceive and read people according to "facial types."[41] At the same time as photography's "truth telling" functions were being embraced, early twentieth-century photographers such as Alfred Stieglitz were making claims for photography's status as art. Angela's painting neatly unites these impulses toward art, truth, and typology, and Fauset's celebration of Angela's work provides a basis for recognizing photography's importance as African-American artists seek ways to "do justice" to their subjects. Indeed, Fauset's novel offers a strikingly apt argument for integrating VanDerZee's work into current accounts of the aesthetic and political debates that shaped the Harlem Renaissance, as his photography addresses issues of mimesis, fantasy, and racial identity.

Angela's painting, however, does not depict African-American subjects, though Fauset notes that the other scholarship goes to an African-American student, Miss Powell, for her painting "A Street in Harlem" (334). At this critical juncture the novel's plot intersects with Du Bois's "Criteria of Negro Art," for in that lecture Du Bois describes "a colored woman in Chicago who is a great musician" who "would like to study at Fontainebleau" but who is prohibited because of race (295). While no direct reference is made to Du Bois's lecture here, Miss Powell's scholarship is indeed rescinded because of her race. As a result Angela is forced to confront her own betrayal of her racial origins, and she publicly reveals her own racial status in protest. Here art and racial politics neatly converge, for Angela's experiences as an artist help to compel her to accept her own racial heritage, while in turn she can use those artistic talents to promote the vision of racial progress that Du Bois presents.

Earlier in the novel, Fauset effectively announces the connection between Angela's art and Du Bois's essay with the cameo appearance of the esteemed black leader "Van Meier," whom Angela hears give a lecture on the need to develop a "racial pride" that "enables us to find our own beautiful" and to be "content with its own types" (219). As the references to beauty and "types" establish, Angela's art could support the development of such a racial pride. She could, in effect, use her talents to discover and draw out the beauty in African-American subjects, as VanDerZee's photographs do. This obvious call to Angela's sense of duty to her race, however, is troubled by an apparent demand for personal sacrifice in pursuing racial solidarity. When Miss Powell refuses to contest her unjust treatment, Angela understands that she submits "so she could have something left in her to devote to her art. You can't fight and create at the same time." As Angela sees it "the matter of blood seems nothing compared with individuality, character, living" (354). For Angela, "individuality" and "living" are entwined with her own personal rather than racial beauty, and her ability to enjoy the privileges and pleasures her appearance brings. Yet even as Angela pits "blood" against "individuality," the novel traces the process by which her own talents and desires come to correspond with the need for a new, racially conscious vision of beauty. With Angela's growing sense of "Truth and Justice," her emphasis on "character" and "living" come to match gracefully with Du Bois's vision of a black artist without requiring her to give up her ambitions. The novel's fairy tale ending even reunites her with the man she loves, a fellow artist, who (through improbable circumstances) has gotten engaged to Angela's sister. Despite these obstacles, once Angela admits her African-American heritage and embarks on her career as an artist, she is rewarded with the reappearance of her noble lover, who intends "to devote himself to REAL ART" (143).

This reconciliation occurs in Paris, the global capital not only of art, but also of fashion and style, as Fauset's novel reminds us. The final scene finds Angela supported by an art scholarship and comfortably ensconced in a fashionable world far from New York. She wakes on Christmas morning after a party, so sleepy that she is "barely able to toss aside her pretty dress" (378). A maid enters to tell her that she has a "package" waiting for her. This elegant "gift" turns out to be Angela's beloved, whom Angela's sister has sent to Paris after realizing her own love for a different suitor. Angela finds her lover waiting for her "searching about in his pockets, slapping his vest, pulling out keys and handkerchiefs," and he jokes that "[t]here ought to be a tag on me somewhere." Clothes, purchases, and guilty pleasures abound in this unlikely and romantic resolution, in which Angela's newfound happiness is expressed as an ability to consume the objects and people whom she desires. Angela has gone from a mere fashion illustrator to an artist and in this final scene she becomes the central figure in a fashionable tableau that befits a VanDerZee photograph. Yet, at the same time, the ending's air of fantasy and sentimentality emphasizes the difficulties that Fauset faces in describing a black woman artist who can at once pursue her personal desires and fulfill a Du Boisian vision of the artist. Fauset's improbable ending struggles to accommodate the imperative for women and artists to relinquish personal desire to collective purpose, while Fauset also refuses to belittle feminine pleasure in dress and fashion. In turn, Fauset (like VanDerZee) invites her readers to delight in the vicarious consumption of fashion, which Du Bois seemingly eschewed. While accepting Du Bois's call for an "Art" that will draw upon "Truth and Justice," Fauset struggles toward different ways of meeting "the Criteria of Negro Art." In doing so, she reveals neglected connections between fashion and fiction, dress and redress.

Like Fauset, VanDerZee's work attempts a reconciliation between personal desires and a sense of duty. With his elaborate staging and emphasis on glamour, his images are at once an invitation to indulge in fantasy and a way of participating in a collective project of revising conceptions of African-American life. In such photographs as *Before the Night Out*, VanDerZee offers up a vision of "having it all"—pleasure, romance, and

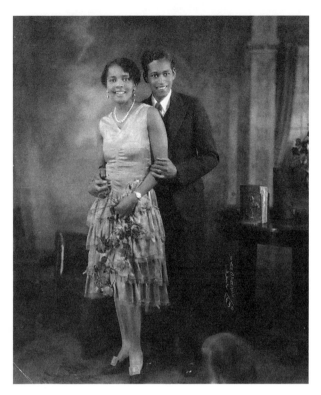

Figure 8.4 James VanDerZee (1886–1983). *Before the Night Out,* 1930. *Courtesy of Donna Mussenden VanDerZee.* (Plate 12.)

respectability—which resonates with *Plum Bun*'s unlikely ending and is supported by the fantasy of fashion (figure 8.4). *Before the Night Out* shows a young, stylishly dressed couple posed in VanDerZee's studio. VanDerZee has hand-colored parts of the girl's dress, as well as her cheeks and lips, the flowers, and a bit of the backdrop beside her. With the image and his manipulations, VanDerZee generates a fictional narrative in which he invites the reader to indulge, while emphasizing the constructedness of this scene. The photograph's date, 1930, underscores the wistfulness of this vision, as the stock market crash of October 1929 marked the beginning of the end of Harlem's days as a destination for pleasure-seekers on their "night out." This belatedness and nostalgia is captured in the girl's dress, for the hemline and tiered skirt were the height of fashion in 1928–1929. At the moment of its creation, then, the photograph is already an image not only of "what has been" (as Barthes says), but what *never* has been. At the same time, the photograph—like Fauset's fiction—is resolutely forward looking. As an image to be circulated among family members and perhaps as a calendar illustration, it celebrates forms of African-American life that are not so much in the past as they are not yet fully realized. In this sense, the photograph offers the same promise of transformation held in the girl's slightly outdated dress.

Fauset and VanDerZee's use of romance and investment in the world of fashion help to explain why their work has not been central to scholarship on the Harlem Renaissance. Yet through their engagement with dress and fantasy, these artists imagine the potential for pleasure, independence, and change in the lives of African-American women. In Harlem in the 1920s and 1930s, racial politics further complicated what Ellen Bayuk Rosenman describes elsewhere in this volume as fashion's "double bind": "On the one hand, dressing well was declared to be women's 'duty,' their contribution to the pleasures of society. Yet at the same time, a woman who took this duty too seriously, or discharged it too successfully, was charged with vanity."[42] In the midst of debates about how best to portray African-Americans, women's "duty" was not only to contribute to "the pleasures of society" but also to support the collective strivings of "the race." At the same time, women who took this duty "too seriously" were open not only to charges of vanity, but also a lack of racial pride. Fauset and VanDerZee attempt to loosen this double bind through their particular hybrid aesthetic, which draws on conventions of romance to depict modern African-American life. Through their use of fantasy, these artists try to imagine fashion as a resource instead of a constraint in negotiating the conditions of modernity. The ambition and limits of their vision underscore fashion's paradoxical association with transformation and futurity as well as with conformity and the return of the old. Their work establishes fashion as a rich symbol and metaphor through which to understand the possibilities and constraints of modern life for African-American women.

Notes

1. W. E. B. Du Bois, "Criteria of Negro Art," *Crisis* (October 1926): 296.
2. Henry Louis Gates, Jr., "The Trope of a New Negro and the Reconstruction of the Image of the Black," *Representations* 24 (Autumn 1988), 148.
3. For a recent discussion on race and portraiture, see Richard J. Powell, *Cutting a Figure: Fashioning Black Portraiture* (Chicago: University of Chicago Press, 2009).
4. See, for example, Hazel Carby, *Reconstructing Womanhood: The Emergence of the Afro-American Woman Novelist* (New York: Oxford University Press, 1987) and Cheryl Wall, *Women of the Harlem Renaissance* (Bloomington: Indiana University Press, 1995).
5. Cherene Sherrard-Johnson, *Portraits of the New Negro Woman: Visual and Literary Culture in the Harlem Renaissance* (New Brunswick: Rutgers University Press, 2007).
6. For studies of the politics of African-American beauty culture in the 1910s through 1930s (including critiques of African-American women's interest in fash-

ion) see Kathy Peiss, *Hope in a Jar: The Making of America's Beauty Culture* (New York: Metropolitan Books, 1998) and Davarian Baldwin, *Chicago's New Negroes: Modernity, the Great Migration, and Black Urban Life* (Chapel Hill: University of North Carolina Press, 2007). For discussions of the depictions of African-American women in *Crisis*, see Caroline Goeser, *Picturing the New Negro: Harlem Renaissance Print Culture and Modern Black Identity* (Lawrence: University Press of Kansas, 2007).

7. For a recent discussion of how this intersects with fashion practices in modernity, see Liz Conor, *The Spectacular Modern Woman: Feminine Visibility in the 1920s* (Bloomington: Indiana University Press, 2004).

8. On visual art in the Renaissance, see Mary Ann Calo, *Distinction and Denial: Race, Nation, and the Critical Construction of the African-American Artist, 1920–1940* (Ann Arbor: University of Michigan Press, 2007) and Sherrard-Johnson, *Portraits of the New Negro Woman*. On illustrations, including images of fashionable women in African-American periodicals, see Goeser, *Picturing the New Negro*. On the intersection of image and text in African-American periodicals, see Anne Elizabeth Carroll, *Word, Image, and the New Negro: Representation and Identity in the Harlem Renaissance* (Bloomington: Indiana University Press, 2005).

9. For a discussion of the narrative dimension of VanDerZee's works, see Deborah Willis-Braithwaite, "They Knew Their Names," *VanDerZee, Photographer: 1886–1983* (New York: Abrams, 1993); and Kobena Mercer, *James Vanderzee 55* (New York: Phaidon, 2003).

10. For a discussion of and a challenge to negative assessments of Fauset's work, see Jane Kuenz, "The Face of America: Performing Race and Nation in Jessie Fauset's *There is Confusion*," *The Yale Journal of Criticism* 12, no. 1 (1999): 89–111. More recent recuperations of Fauset's work include Susan Tomlinson, "Vision to Visionary: The New Negro Woman as Cultural Worker in Jessie Redmon Fauset's *Plum Bun*," *Legacy* 19, no.1 (2002): 90–97; and "An Unwonted Coquetry: The Commercial Seductions of Jessie Fauset's *The Chinaberry Tree*" in *Middlebrow Moderns: Popular American Women Writers of the 1920s*, ed. Lisa Botshon and Meredith Goldsmith (Boston: Northeastern University Press, 2003); Lori Harrison-Kahan, "No Slaves to Fashion: Designing Women in the Fiction of Jessie Fauset and Anzia Yezierska," in *Styling Texts: Dress and Fashion in Literature*, ed. Cynthia Kuhn and Cindy Carlson (Amherst: Cambria Press, 2007); Susan Levison, "Performance and the 'Strange Place' of Jessie Redmon Fauset's *There is Confusion*," *Modern Fiction Studies* 46, no. 4 (Winter 2000): 825–48; Kathleen Pfeiffer, "The Limits of Identity in Jessie Fauset's *Plum Bun*," *Legacy* 18, no. 1 (2001): 79–93; Sharon L. Jones, *Rereading the Harlem Renaissance: Race, Class, and Gender in the Fiction of Jessie Fauset, Zora Neale Hurston, and Dorothy West* (Praeger: Westport, 2002).

11. In interviews later in life, VanDerZee claimed not to have been a supporter of Garvey. James Haskins, *James Van DerZee: The Picture Takin' Man* (New York: Dodd, Mead, 1979).

12. Mercer notes that VanDerZee was a keen observer of the "social world of community-building" developing in Harlem particularly after World War I (8). Mercer, *James Vanderzee*.

13. Georg Simmel, "The Philosophy of Fashion" [1899], in *Simmel on Culture*, ed. David Frisby and Mike Featherstone (London: Sage, 1997): 187–206.

14. Roland Barthes, *Camera Lucida: Reflections on Photography*, trans. Richard Howard (New York: Hill and Wang, 1981), 34. Shawn Michelle Smith notes that Barthes makes these observations when discussing Richard Avedon's 1963 portrait "William Casby, born a slave," and her chapter brilliantly unpacks the racialist logic that underpins Barthes's claims about objectification in photography. Smith, "Race and Reproduction in *Camera Lucida*," in *Photography Degree Zero: Reflections on Roland Barthes's* Camera Lucida, ed. Geoffrey Batchen (Cambridge, MA: MIT Press, 2009), 246.

15. For a discussion of VanDerZee's work for calendars, see Willis-Braithwaite, "They Knew Their Names."

16. For a discussion of Simpson's work in relation to VanDerZee's compositions, see Sara Blair, *Harlem Crossroads: Black Writers and the Photograph in the Twentieth Century* (Princeton: Princeton University Press, 2007).

17. The subjects of VanDerZee's photographs appear to have supplied their own clothing. However, Dawoud Bey has asserted that VanDerZee's studio did have "fine clothes" for patrons to put on if they so chose, and a very few photographs that I have seen do appear to feature the same garments on different people. Bey, "Authoring the Black Image: The Photographs of James VanDerZee," *The James VanDerZee Studio,* ed. Colin Westbrook (The Art Institute of Chicago: Chicago, 2004), 33. For a discussion of VanDerZee's "directorial" approach, see Willis-Braithwaite, "They Knew Their Names."

18. On "thing theory," see Bill Brown, *A Sense of Things: The Object Matter of American Literature* (Chicago: University of Chicago Press, 2003). Feminist theory has long worked to critique this idea of the dematerialized autonomous subject and to expose the way that it establishes a white, male, heterosexual individual as a normative subject. Ilya Parkins has discussed the ways that fashion can aid this feminist project of situating the modern subject in its particular material and cultural conditions. Parkins, *Material Modernity: A Feminist Theory of Modern Fashion* (PhD dissertation, York University, 2005).

19. For a related discussion of the role of dress in constructing African-Americans as subjects of portraiture, see Powell.

20. For discussion of the "Victorian" style of VanDerZee's work, see Willis-Braithwaite, "They Knew Their Names," and Mercer, *James Vanderzee.*

21. Haskins, 87–88.

22. Haskins, 158. When VanDerZee's work was first "discovered" in 1969 as part of the infamous "Harlem on My Mind" exhibition at the Metropolitan Museum, his work was valued as a form of documentation of Harlem life, and the artistic or creative aspects of his work were largely disregarded. More recently critics have analyzed the aesthetic and ideological investments guiding VanDerZee's photography, although some work remains to be done to explore the complexities of his art. For example, in Sara Blair's recent study of African-American writers and photography in the mid-to-late twentieth century, she asserts that later writers and photographers defined themselves in contrast to the "uplift-inflected conventions of Harlem portraiture (exemplified by the commissioned studio work of James VanDerZee)" and others (10). Blair implies a contrast between VanDerZee's narrow vision and the innovation of later photographers. Blair, *Harlem Crossroads.*

23. Mercer, 8–9. Mercer also sees clothing as signifying modernity in contrast to VanDerZee's old-fashioned backdrops.

24. Hughes, *The Big Sea* [1940] (New York: Hill and Wang, 1993), 218.

25. See, for example, Deborah E. McDowell, "The Neglected Dimension of Jessie Redmon Fauset," *Conjuring: Black Women, Fiction, and Literary Tradition*, ed. Marjorie Pryse and Hortense J. Spillers (Bloomington: Indiana University Press, 1985), 86–104; Tomlinson, "Vision to Visionary"; Jones, *Rereading the Harlem Renaissance*.

26. Daylanne K. English, *Unnatural Selections: Eugenics in American Modernism and the Harlem Renaissance* (Chapel Hill: University of North Carolina Press, 2004).

27. In *Three Generations*, the presence of the woman who stands behind the elderly women helps to interrupt the family narrative, which VanDerZee's image creates. Her tentative expression and her position behind the chair underscore the she does not share the striking resemble which the other women display. She may be a sister of the two middle-aged women, but she seems like an unaccounted for outsider, who reminds us of the artificiality of this family grouping.

28. Russ Castronovo, "Beauty Along the Color Line: Lynching, Aesthetics, and the *Crisis*," *Beautiful Democracy: Aesthetics and Anarchy in a Global Era* (Chicago: University of Chicago Press, 2007), 130.

29. For discussions of how this reading has explicitly and implicitly shaped the reception of VanDerZee's work, see Charles Martin, "Implied Texts and the Colors of Photography," *The African Diaspora: African origins and New World Identities*, ed. Isidore Okpewho, Carole Boyce Davies, Ali A. Mazrui (Bloomington: Indiana University Press, 2001), 458; and Richard J. Powell, "Linguists, Poets, and 'Others' on African-American Art," *American Art* 17, no. 1 (Spring 2003): 16–19. For a discussion of readings of Fauset in this vein, see Kuenz, "The Face of America."

30. Du Bois, 297.

31. For a discussion of critiques of beauty culture as imitation, see Peiss. Nella Larsen's *Quicksand* features a member of Harlem's black elite who professes that she hates white people even as she "aped their clothes, their manners, and their gracious ways of living." Larsen, *Quicksand*, ed. Thadious Davis (New York: Penguin, 2002), 51.

32. Barthes, 43. For an analysis of Barthes's racialist logic, see Smith, Race and Reproduction."

33. Critics have often noted how the association between consumer culture and whiteness inflects Nella Larsen's novels *Quicksand* and *Passing*. See, for example, Goldsmith, "Shopping to Pass, Passing to Shop: Consumer Self-Fashioning in the Fiction of Nella Larsen," in *Middlebrow Moderns: Popular American Women Writers of the 1920*, ed. Lisa Botshon and Meredith Goldsmith (Boston: Northeastern University Press, 2003), 269; and Alys Eve Weinbaum, "Racial Masquerade: Consumption and Contestation of American Modernity," *The Modern Girl Around the World: Consumption, Modernity, and Globalization*, ed. The Modern Girl Around the World Research Group (Alys Eve Weinbaum, Lynn M. Thomas, Priti Ramamurthy, Uta G. Poiger, Madeleine Yue Don, and Tani E. Barlow) (Durham: Duke University Press, 2008), 120–46. For a discussion of early twentieth-century critiques of African-American beauty culture as imitative, see Peiss.

34. Tomlinson, "Vision to Visionary," 240.

35. Tomlinson, 241.

36. Du Bois, "Criteria of Negro Art," 292.

37. Jessie Fauset, *Plum Bun*, intro by Deborah E. McDowell (London: Pandora Press, 1985), 13. All quotations refer to this edition and subsequent page numbers will be cited parenthetically in the text.

38. Du Bois, "Criteria of Negro Art," 296.

39. For recent discussions of what is at stake with the aesthetic experiments of *Fire!!!*, see Michael L. Cobb, "Insolent Racing, Rough Narrative: The Harlem Renaissance's Impolite Queers," *Callaloo* 23, no. 1 (2000): 328–51; and Stephen Knadler, "Sweetback Style: Wallace Thurman and a Queer Harlem Renaissance," *Modern Fiction Studies* 48, no. 4 (Winter 2002): 899–936.

40. For a discussion of Fauset's allusions to the Fourteenth Street School, see Tomlinson, "Vision to Visionary."

41. Walter Benjamin, "Little History of Photography," *Selected Writings Volume 2, 1927–1934*, trans. Rodney Livingston and others, ed. Michael W. Jennings, Howard Eiland, and Gary Smith (Cambridge, MA: Belknap Press, 1999), 520.

42. Rosenman, 155.

9

"MORE THAN A GARMENT"

Edna Ferber and the Fashioning of
Transnational Identity

In an 1896 speech in which he argued for the drastic curtailment of immigration to the United States, Senator Henry Cabot Lodge voiced the fear that the unrestricted acceptance of foreigners would effect "a great and perilous change in the very fabric of our race." While Lodge addressed the negative economic impact of immigration, calling "low, unskilled labor . . . the most deadly enemy of the American wage earner," his main concern was the danger posed "to the quality of our citizenship."[1] As Lodge's warnings illustrate, the increase in immigration at the turn of the century led to a rise in nativism, which reached its height in the 1920s with the passage of immigration quotas and the Johnson-Reed Act of 1924. Like most nativists, Lodge relied upon notions of scientific racism, fueled by the eugenics movement, and insisted on inherent distinctions between racial groups. His metaphor of race as a fabric, however, potentially undermines such essentialist claims. In this essay, I address how this material metaphor, originating in the discourses of nativism and scientific racism, is taken up in cultural pluralism as a loophole in nativist thought. I do so by mining an untapped source, the fiction of Jewish-American writer Edna Ferber, whose early work, published in the second decade of the twentieth century, centered on ethnic female protagonists employed in the fashion industry. Placing Ferber's fiction in the context of turn-of-the-twentieth-century immigration debates, this chapter builds upon Ilya Parkins and Elizabeth Sheehan's notion of fashion as an "integrative medium." In the introduction to this book, Parkins and Sheehan describe fashion's ability to bridge divides between public and private, intimate and spectacular, individual and collective, and material and conceptual. I expand upon their definition to demonstrate that fashion similarly allows for the interweaving of ethnic and class as well as gender differences and thus holds out the promise of a democratic, pluralist ideal.

The Fabric of Our Race

Maintaining the biological inferiority of immigrants, nativists continually expressed concerns that foreigners would manipulate their material environment in order to imitate, blend in with, and ultimately contaminate the American race. In Madison Grant's 1916 *The Passing of the Great Race*, for example, the author warns that the new strain of immigrants would "elbow" the American "out of his own home" and ultimately lead to his "extermina[tion]." Like many nativists, Grant viewed the influx of Jews from Eastern Europe as an exemplary evil. They "adopt the language of the native American," Grant wrote of Jewish immigrants, "they wear his clothes, they steal his name, and they are beginning to take his women, but they seldom adopt his religion or understand his ideals."[2] German ethnographer Richard Andree articulated similar ideas in his study of the Jewish Diaspora: "Even when he adopts the language, dress, habits, and customs of the people among whom he lives, he still remains everywhere the same. All he adopts is but a cloak, under which the eternal Hebrew survives; he is the same in his facial features, in the structure of his body, his temperament, his character."[3] By using the "cloak" to refer inclusively to "language, dress, habits, and customs," Andree reveals that the immigrant's ability to obscure his racial difference through clothes was a particular source of anxiety. While Andree referred to essential physiognomic and personality traits that remain the same despite the donning of a "cloak," sociologist E. A. Ross suggested that clothing utterly fails to conceal difference when he argued that the New World should close its gates to foreigners. According to Ross's *The Old World in the New* (1914), immigrants continue to "look out of place in black clothes and stiff collar, since clearly they belong in skins, in wattled huts at the close of the Great Ice Age."[4] For Ross, proper clothing may function as a marker of civilization, but it cannot conceal the primitivism of the immigrant. As scientific racism attempted to ascribe Jewish difference to the body, clothing—which marked the somewhat tenuous boundary between the bodily self and the environment beyond it—became highly contested territory in debates about the racialization of Jewish immigrants.

While nativists often used the rhetoric of clothes to express fears of racial contamination, their opponents also turned to figurative language in order to imagine a more inclusive nation. The popular metaphor of the melting pot, for example, offered an idealistic image of a nation in which immigrants were easily assimilated and Americanized, their differences made innocuous when tempered. "America is God's Crucible, the great Melting-Pot where all the races of Europe are melting and reforming" to produce "the real American," declaims a character in British playwright Israel Zangwill's *The Melting-Pot*.[5] For advocates of the melting pot, the ability to transform oneself through dress was a triumphant spectacle rather than a source of anxiety. In the 1910s, Henry Ford's immigrant employees who were enrolled in his English Language School participated in graduation ceremonies in which they descended into an oversized papier-mâché cauldron wearing their national peasant garb, were stirred by ladles wielded by their teachers, and then reemerged clothed in American dress, waving the stars and stripes.[6] This dramatic scene conflated the glories of mass production with the successful Americanization of immigrants, promising a leveling of the playing field through the mechanization of workers and consumer goods.

For many intellectuals of the time, the nativist and melting pot visions, though seemingly opposed to each other, were equally problematic. These intellectuals argued instead for a pluralistic society, welcoming immigrants with the expectation that they would retain, rather than renounce, their ethnic and cultural differences. In a direct response to E.A. Ross, philosopher Horace Kallen published a 1915 essay entitled "Democracy versus the Melting-Pot." Defining "Americanization" as "the adoption of English speech, of American clothes and manners, of the American attitude in politics," Kallen developed an extended musical metaphor when he envisioned an alternative to the melting pot. He conceived of each ethnic group as an "instrument" in an orchestra, working together to create a "symphony of civilization." As each group contributed its distinct "timbre and tonality," "the range and variety of the harmonies may become wider and richer and more beautiful."[7] By drawing his analogy from the realm of high art, Kallen suggested that the different ethnic groups have their own contributions to make to civilization, and thus he countered Ross's view of immigrants as uncivilized and primitive.

In his 1916 essay "Trans-National America," philosopher Randolph Bourne articulated similar ideas, rejecting the alchemistic and culinary metaphors of the melting pot while appropriating the nativists' use of textile imagery. Answering depictions of immigrants as "masses of aliens, waiting to be 'assimilated,' waiting to be melted down into the indistinguishable dough of Anglo-Saxonism," Bourne instead described them as "threads of living and potent cultures, blindly striving to weave themselves into a novel international nation, the first the world has seen." In effect, Bourne responds to and reverses Lodge's metaphor with which I opened. America becomes a "unique sociological fabric," "not a nationality, but a trans-nationality, a weaving back and forth, with . . . other lands, of many threads of all sizes and colors." Speaking against nativists and proponents of the melting pot, Bourne warned against "attempts to thwart this weaving, or to dye the fabric any one color, or disentangle the threads of the strands."[8] Rather than weakening the "fabric of [the] race," as Lodge proposed, Bourne maintained that immigrants would combine to create a superior cloth knit from varied strands. Like Kallen, Bourne resolved the tensions between assimilation and cultural preservation by imagining "richer and more beautiful" entities constructed from a plurality of differences.

There has been, to date, little discussion of the way the various discourses surrounding immigration in early twentieth-century America drew on the language of textiles and apparel. Yet psychological and economic tracts on fashion and dress proliferated from the turn of the century through the 1920s as the rise of mass production occasioned a boom in the garment industry. In perhaps the most famous example, *The Theory of the Leisure Class* (1899), economist Thorstein Veblen speculated that the increasingly industrialized production of dress would have a dramatic impact on socioeconomic divisions because ready-to-wear clothes made it possible for the working classes to imitate the styles of the upper classes. The wide availability of consumer goods transformed workers into consumers and, in effect, allowed the lower classes to pose as something they were not. In turn, according to Veblen, this accelerated "the phenomenon of changing fashions," as the upper classes sought to maintain the signs of their socio-economic superiority.[9]

Veblen's work has proved an important point of reference for feminist theorists of fashion, since gender plays a crucial role in his theory of "conspicuous consumption," the notion that the purchase and display of clothes and other consumer goods could be used to signal economic and social status. Through dress, women of the leisure class became ornaments to mark the monetary value of the men who saw them as property. Leading feminist intellectual Charlotte Perkins Gilman rehearsed Veblen's theories to emphasize clothes as a factor in sex distinction in her own statement on dress, titled *The Dress of Women*, which appeared in her monthly journal *The Forerunner* in 1915. While holding to Veblen's class-based explanation of fashion changes, Gilman also emphasized the role that dress plays in the social construction of gender, arguing that the differences between the sexes are due to attire rather than biology. Gilman contended that the so-called "physical limitations of women" are "due to the limitations of their clothes and of the conduct supposed to belong to them." In one example, she writes, "The mincing twittering gait, supposed to be 'feminine,' is only 'skirtine'—it has nothing to do with sex."[10]

As feminist reformers such as Gilman drew attention to the restrictions imposed by dress, fashion design followed suit. According to fashion historian Valerie Steele, the years between 1906 and 1916 marked a revolution for women's fashion. Beginning to blur the sex distinction that troubled Gilman, styles changed from the Victorian corset to simpler and more functional modernist designs. After World War I, women designers such as Chanel looked to men's clothes for inspiration not only because of the comfort and practicality they provided, but also because of the independence and power they represented. Chanel's designs became emblematic of the shift in women's fashion, and, as a self-made businesswoman who used fashion to reinvent herself, the designer became as iconic as her designs. Despite being likened to a man due to her sharp business sense, Chanel insisted on her femininity, and her clothes were similarly renowned for bringing together seemingly oppositional elements.[11]

The feminist literature on fashion has mostly failed to take into account the ways that gender and class intersect with race and ethnicity, despite increasing critical attention to intersectionality within the broader field of feminist studies.[12] Given that immigrants composed the majority of the urban working class in turn-of-the-century America, it behooves us to revisit Veblen's economic critique in order to read it as ethnically coded. In late nineteenth- and early twentieth-century America, it was typically immigrant women who developed a special relationship to clothes as both workers and consumers. In particular, in the 1880s and 1890s, the arrival of large numbers of Jewish immigrants from Eastern Europe coincided with the expansion of the garment industry, especially in the area of women's apparel, and these immigrants became the main source of cheap labor in the rapidly developing textile and apparel industries. Many found work in factories, feeding the demand for mass-produced clothes, while members of a more select group were employed as salesgirls in that relatively new urban institution, the department store. Unlike other industries, the fashion industry was not sex-segregated, since the manufacture of clothes was seen as a trade for both men and women. Jewish communities often encouraged women to participate in the domestic economy as breadwinners, and immigrant women came armed with skills they had acquired working in factories and workshops in the Old World, where many had been trained as dressmakers and seamstresses.[13]

While Veblen, Gilman, and other theorists of fashion and consumer culture have focused on the ways that dress creates gender and class distinctions, the fiction of early twentieth-century Jewish women writers such as Edna Ferber and Anzia Yezierska, as well as that of African-American writers such as Jessie Fauset, employed dress to explore the fashioning of *ethnic* womanhood.[14] Focusing on Ferber's fiction, which was published as the fashion industry was undergoing an experimental phase that served as a transition from Victorian to modern ideals, this essay establishes how the figure of the ethnic working woman operates at the nexus of various discourses surrounding consumerism and class, women and gender, and immigration and ethnicity. Ferber's writing is an apt case study not only because of its subject matter, but also because of its tremendous popularity, especially with a female readership. Beginning with her first novel, *Dawn O'Hara* (1911), a partially autobiographical tale of a female journalist, Ferber testifies to the changes taking place in gender roles during the early decades of the twentieth century by documenting the emergence of the New Woman. Ferber went on to seize the national consciousness with the Emma McChesney stories, the wildly popular series following the adventures of a divorced single mother who supports herself and her son by working as a skirt and petticoat saleswoman. Heralded as a "new type" and lauded as the first businesswoman of American fiction when she made her literary debut in 1911, Emma McChesney enjoyed a five-year run in the pages of *American Magazine* and *Cosmopolitan*.[15] Much like designer-businesswoman Chanel, Ferber's protagonist champions products that capture the gender and class ambivalences faced by middle-class women as they became wage earners outside the home, increasingly entering the "masculine" public sphere.

Even as her heroine's last name signals her Irish background, Ferber largely suppressed the issue of ethnicity in the Emma McChesney stories. However, in two pieces of fiction Ferber published after retiring Emma, she confronted ethnic identity head-on. Ferber's 1918 short story "The Girl Who Went Right" and her 1917 autobiographical novel, *Fanny Herself*, also take the apparel industry as their backdrop, featuring protagonists who make their livings as sellers of clothes. Both works involve Jewish working women who "pass," hiding their ethnic backgrounds for the sake of their employment. In emphasizing the effect of ready-made clothes on economic and gender divisions, Ferber's narratives address anxieties described in Veblen's *The Theory of the Leisure Class* that the rise of mass production would threaten class barriers, but, through the trope of passing, they also acknowledge the intertwining of class status with ethnic identity. My readings of these two fictions illustrate how Veblen's ideas were echoed in nativist fears that ethnic "others" would infiltrate Ameri-

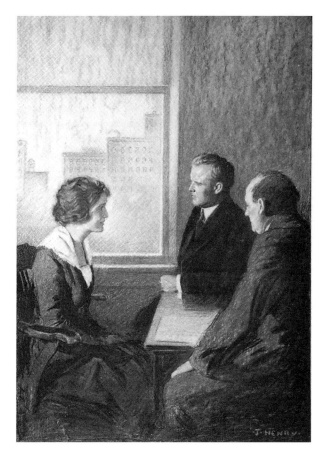

Figure 9.1 J. Henry, "'Now, Miss Brandeis, what's the trouble with the Haynes-Cooper infants' wear department?'" Illustration in Edna Ferber's *Fanny Herself* (Frederick A. Stokes Company, 1917). *Samuel Paley Library, Temple University.*

can citizenship—fears that necessitated the policing of corporeal and national borders.

In the section that follows, I examine how "The Girl Who Went Right" functions as a cautionary tale about the dangers of erasing one's past, specifically by using fashion as a site to critique the ideology of the melting pot. Moving on to analyze *Fanny Herself*, I demonstrate that Ferber does not simply condemn fashion as a symptom of problematic conformity, but also employs its materiality to construct a pluralistic alternative to assimilationism. I conclude by showing how the protagonist of *Fanny Herself* comes to fashion a hybrid model of identity, one in which supposedly incompatible strands—femininity and masculinity, Jewishness and Americanness, the working and the leisure class—have the potential to be woven together to create enriched wholes. Ferber's vision is not necessarily radical; she does not propose a wholesale rejection of gender roles, for example, and her characters, even when offered the opportunity, decline to align themselves explicitly with the first-wave feminist movement.

However, in employing the medium of fashion to frame and portray modern women who construct themselves in complex, multiple, and often shifting ways, her fiction works against the notion that one can be forced into a pigeonhole of identity.

The Girl Who Went White

Just as nativists tended to see Jews as a particularly pernicious breed of immigrants, pluralists such as Kallen and Bourne saw Jews as exemplary in quite another sense. In their ability to reconcile national differences by simultaneously adopting American values and retaining their own culture, Jews became emblematic of cultural pluralism and trans-nationality. Having authored a version of his philosophy of Americanism titled "The Jew and Trans-National America," Bourne stated, "It is not the Jew who sticks proudly to the faith of his fathers and boasts of that venerable culture of his who is dangerous to America, but the Jew who has lost the Jewish fire and become a mere elementary grasping animal."[16] In "Democracy versus the Melting-Pot," Kallen prized the ability of Jewish immigrants to develop a distinct culture on American soil, describing them as both "the most eagerly American of the immigrant groups" and "the most autonomous and self-conscious in spirit and culture."[17]

In her earliest works of fiction, *Dawn O'Hara* and the Emma McChesney stories, Ferber represented the average working woman in Irish protagonists whose ethnic identities were mostly inconsequential to their stories. Yet Ferber, the daughter of a Hungarian immigrant father and a second-generation German-Jewish mother, considered her own ethnic background to be formative to her identity and to her career as a writer. She described her first autobiographical installment, *A Peculiar Treasure*, as "the story of an American Jewish family in the past half-century, and as such ... really a story about America which I know and love."[18] In *Fanny Herself* and "The Girl Who Went Right," narratives that followed on the heels of Kallen and Bourne's writings, Ferber not only transformed her New Women heroines into Jews, but also made her characters' Jewishness a crucial component of the plots. Occluding and then reclaiming their ethnic affiliations, Ferber's Jewish characters become representative of pluralist ideals in a way that her Irish characters were not. Like Kallen and Bourne, Ferber viewed Jews as exemplary of a national ideology in which one could claim patriotic citizenship without forsaking one's ethnic and cultural heritage.

Set against the growth of mass production taking place in the early twentieth-century apparel industry, both "The Girl Who Went Right" and *Fanny Herself* employ the material metaphor of fashion to problematize the imitativeness of immigrant assimilation. While Veblen wrote of the ability of ready-made clothes to erode class differences and nativists expressed apprehension that immigration would threaten racial purity, "The Girl Who Went Right" unites these twin fears. It demonstrates how the body of the woman—as a showcase for conspicuous consumption and a vehicle for racial amalgamation—menaces carefully established boundaries of class and race. Furthermore, the immigrant working woman at the center of Ferber's fiction presents an additional threat to gender norms in challenging the notion of separate spheres. Through its protagonist's initial rejection and subsequent reclamation of her Jewish identity, Ferber's story moralistically critiques the immigrant's attempt to mimic white Anglo-Saxon femininity, but encapsulated in this critique is an exposé of whiteness and femininity as unachievable, and not necessarily desirable, ideals.

"The Girl Who Went Right" opens with its protagonist, Rachel Wiletzky, changing her name to Ray Willets in order to secure a job as a salesgirl at a department store. This Americanized name assists Rachel in persuading the superintendent to try her out as a shopgirl, but Rachel's shortening of her name also comes to signify how she has excised part of herself so as not to be seen as an outsider in America. Forsaking her Jewish identity to worship in the house of fashion, the newly invented Ray Willets hopes to resist further the image of the coarse and uncultured immigrant woman when she expresses her preference for selling lingerie. By surrounding herself with soft and silky undergarments, Rachel intends to underscore her feminine attributes and disassociate further from her ethnic background. Describing her reverence for a peignoir that she is called upon to model for a customer, Rachel reflects, "It was more than a garment. It represented in her mind a new standard of all that was beautiful and exquisite and desirable."[19] By declaring the nightgown "more than a garment," Rachel invests it with symbolic value, acknowledging that dress has the ability to testify to one's status in American society. In this case, the luxurious lingerie operates as a signifier of leisure-class femininity, which is at odds with Rachel's working-class immigrant identity. That Rachel's entry into this stylish world coincides with her decision to obscure her heritage demonstrates how fashion serves as a metaphor for self-fashioning in the Jewish immigrant experience.

Jewish immigrants may have used dress to construct their new identities, endowing clothing with the meaning that made it "more than a garment," but they also symbolically conceived of their pasts as garments to be discarded, thus replacing one material identity with another. The protagonist of "The Girl Who Went Right" was certainly not alone in drawing on the historical conditions of labor to imagine the process of Americanization through the language of clothes. Jewish immigrant Mary Antin, for example, used a similar analogy in her 1912 autobiography, *The Promised Land*. Imagining her prior life as "a heavy garment that clings to your limbs when you ... run," Antin endeavors to "release" herself "from the folds of the clinging past."[20]

As the adjectives "clinging" and "heavy" suggest, the past may be no more than a garment, but this does not necessarily make it easy to discard. While dress signals the capacity for reinvention, it also serves to reveal the difficulties of erasing the past. In "The Girl Who Went Right," Rachel's job is constantly threatened by her inability to acquire the proper attire. In one scene, for example, when Rachel removes the robe she was modeling for a customer, she reveals a rip under her arm, an infraction in her appearance that subjects her to the scolding of Miss Jevne, head of the lingerie department. The tear may evoke Andree's description of the "eternal Hebrew" who survives beneath the "cloak" he wears to blend in, but it is also significant that the imperfection, which serves as the marker of difference, appears in Rachel's shirtwaist, itself an article of clothing. In the words of Homi Bhabha, Rachel's mimicry might be described as "almost the same, but not quite"—or, as Bhabha expands on his formulation, "almost the same, but not white."[21] Rachel's inadequate mimicry continues to place her job in jeopardy. When the salesgirls are instructed to wear gowns to work, Rachel fails to purchase the requisite uniform because her family needs her income to care for a sick child. In return for putting her "own folks" before fashion (68), she is temporarily demoted to selling kitchenware. The domestic space of the kitchen is deemed more suitable for a woman of her class and ethnicity unless her identity can be effectively disguised through dress.

"The Girl Who Went Right" links Rachel's imitation of white American identity to the imitations of high fashion that were the subject of Veblen's caustic commentary. Desperate for salesgirls, Miss Jevne calls Rachel back to the lingerie section and agrees to lend her a black gown. Observing Rachel's new frock, one of the other salesgirls notes that it "looks just like one of our eighteen-dollar models" (70) and wonders if Rachel had copied it. As Nan Enstad illustrates in her study of working women at the turn of the century, "department store workers were infamous for learning the styles from the clothing they sold."[22] But when the salesgirls gush over the newest model of lingerie, once again suggesting that Rachel might be able to take one home in order to create a reproduction, Rachel's contempt for the garment is evident: "That's just a cheap skirt. Only twelve-fifty. Machine-made lace. Imitation embroidery—" (70). At this moment, Rachel breaks off, realizing her own susceptibility to the superficiality that surrounds her. Here Ferber seems to take a page out of Veblen's book: "With few and inconsequential exceptions, we all find a costly handwrought article of apparel much preferable, in point of beauty and of serviceability, to a less expensive imitation of it, however cleverly the spurious article may imitate the costly original. . . . The offensive object may be so close an imitation as to defy any but the closest scrutiny; and yet so soon as the counterfeit is detected, its aesthetic value, and its commercial value as well, declines precipitately."[23] When applied to Rachel herself, Veblen's words echo nativist fears that racial mingling would allow foreigners to impersonate Americans.

As the title of the story indicates, Ferber's heroine eventually tires of her deception and realizes the error of her ways. Rachel may attempt to go "white" when she changes her name, but she goes "right" at the end of the story, which concludes with an affirmation of her Jewish identity, as she once again declares herself "Rachel Wiletzky." Once a fervent believer in fashion's transformative potential, Rachel becomes increasingly disillusioned as she encounters the phoniness of the high-fashion world that her falsehood about her name allows her to enter. She comes to realize that the life she initially saw as more "desirable," and more real, than her own is itself built upon fakery. While Rachel's self-naming is an attempt to cover up her ethnic heritage, the fashion industry concerns itself with the construction of femininity; after all, it would not exist were femininity purely natural. Indicating how class is closely intertwined with gender and ethnicity, Rachel's rejection of the materialistic values she has adopted coincides with her rejection of her own aspirations to whiteness and her refusal to participate fully in the "mas(s)querade," in Tania Modleski's pun, that is femininity.[24] At the end of the story, she asks to be transferred back to kitchen utensils and household goods, where she does not "have to tell a woman how graceful and charming she's going to look while she's working the washing machine" (69). Rachel has come to resent the lies she must tell in the lingerie department in order to perpetuate the greater lie about femininity, but her protest remains contained within the confines of consumer culture, resulting only in the replacement of one feminine and domestic space for another.

Rachel's avowal of her former identity may also appear to uphold Jewishness as the inescapable identity beneath the cloak, even as "The Girl Who Went Right" differs from nativist claims of immutable difference by making its heroine's reclamation of her heritage a matter of pride rather than inferiority. But Ferber's text does not simply affirm Rachel's

Jewish identity as her "true" self. Instead, it troubles the very notion of authenticity in two related ways: first, through its representation of Jewishness as a category of identity that eludes concrete definition; and second, through its continued reliance on material metaphors.

In "The Girl Who Went Right," Jewishness operates to confuse authenticity because it cannot be easily defined. While there may be little ambiguity about whether or not Rachel is Jewish, there is ambiguity about what Jewishness *is* and thus what it is that makes one Jewish. In the story, there is not a single direct mention of the word "Jew." Instead, the reader is left to draw her own conclusion about Rachel's identity, based on clues such as her name, her "ghetto voice" (59), a reference to a Talmud-studying ancestor, and perhaps even the knowledge that Ferber herself was Jewish. Because of an almost complete absence of references to religion or religious practice, Rachel's Jewish identity is not a spiritual one. Instead, her identity is most clearly defined in racial terms, as when the text describes her "latent dramatic force" as a "heritage of her race" (60). Yet, with this very description, the story challenges whether racial traits are dependable signs of identity, since Rachel's only ascribed racial quality is her ability to perform. As scholars such as Sander Gilman and Daniel Itzkovitz have shown, Jews were thought to have an innate talent for mimicry, which made them especially adaptable to assimilation, since they were able to blend in with any group of people. In this association of Jews with performativity, Jewishness thus comes to symbolize the paradoxes and slipperiness of identity—a lack of fixity that, while threatening to nativists, could also prove liberating.[25]

Although the text continually draws attention to Rachel's difference from those around her, it positions her not only as distinct from the white majority, but also from other immigrants since she is unmarked by stereotypically Jewish attributes. Upon Rachel's first appearance in his office, the superintendent takes note of her beauty, commenting that she "was as much out of place among the preceding one hundred and seventy-eight bloodless, hollow-chested, stoop-shouldered applicants as a sunflower would be in a patch of dank white fungi" (58). Rachel's brightness is contrasted with "dank" whiteness, a description that, unexpectedly, gives whiteness negative connotations. Rachel continues to defy all attempts to pin down her identity, resisting explanations that rely on biology as well as environment. When she is asked to fill out an application form explaining why she is leaving her current job to work at the department store, she protests, "How can I say on a blank that I'm leaving because I want to be where real people are? What chance has a girl got over there on the West Side? I'm different. . . . I don't know why but I am.

Look at my face! Where should I get red cheeks from? From not having enough to eat half the time and sleeping three in a bed?" (60).

Like the paradoxical belief that a tendency toward the dramatic can serve as proof of one's essential and authentic Jewishness, this passage illuminates several contradictory claims about identity. The text may describe Rachel's "dramatic force" as a racial quality, but she also claims difference from other Jews, especially due to her physical appearance. Rachel deconstructs the divide between nature and nurture when she asks where her red cheeks come from: the implication is that they cannot be the result of the Jewish heritage the text has just alluded to, since Jews were traditionally associated with darker coloring, nor can they be result of her poor living conditions. Even as Rachel continually sets others straight about their assumptions of nurture, the text refuses to come down on the side of nature; instead, it refuses any simple explanation for Rachel's appearance, just as Jewish performativity blurs the line between construction and essentialism. These contradictions challenge the reliability of signs to identify one's "real" race and insist upon the indeterminacy of difference—which is why the text resists using the word "Jew."

As the story proceeds to engage in a mocking commentary on what constitutes authenticity, the realness of gender and the realness of race become inextricable. For example, Rachel contrasts herself to Miss Jevne, whom she holds up as a paragon of femininity:

Of Miss Jevne it might be said that she was real where Ray was artificial, and artificial where Ray was real. Everything that Miss Jevne wore was real. She was as modish as Ray was shabby, as slim as Ray was stocky, as artificially tinted and tinctured as Ray was naturally rosy-cheeked and buxom. It takes real money to buy clothes as real as those worn by Miss Jevne. The soft charmeuse in her graceful gown was real and miraculously draped. The cobweb-lace collar that so delicately traced its pattern against the black background of her gown was real. So was the ripple of lace that cascaded down the front of her blouse. The straight, correct, hideously modern lines of her figure bespoke a real eighteen-dollar corset. Realest of all, there reposed on Miss Jevne's bosom a bar pin of platinum and diamonds—very real diamonds set in a severely plain but very real bar of precious platinum. So if you except Miss Jevne's changeless colour, her artificial smile, her glittering hair and her undulating head-of-the-department walk, you can see that everything about Miss Jevne was as real as money can make one. (62)

Although Ferber's satirical voice clearly mocks Miss Jevne's brand of the real, Rachel herself does not wake to the realization that her boss is all fakery and adornment until the end of the story. The contrast between

Rachel and Miss Jevne is ironic, for what makes Miss Jevne real are her clothes and jewels, while Rachel's own realness is dependent on features such as shape and coloring. The story further complicates categories of identity by implying that Miss Jevne's high-class appearance may be attained at the expense of her ethnic background and her feminine virtue. Because department stores put saleswomen at risk for prostitution, employers preferred to hire women who lived with their families, a question Rachel is asked on her job application.[26] Miss Jevne, Rachel learns, has cut herself off from her family on the West Side in order to live alone— the implication being that she has forsaken both her morals and her heritage, which remains ambiguous, despite the fact that her name begins to spell "Jew" and that she, like Rachel, comes from the West Side of the city. Rachel's climactic change of heart is occasioned by the realization that what Zangwill calls the "real American" is a mass-produced façade and that buying into the ideology of the melting pot involves sacrificing vital aspects of one's cultural heritage and integrity.

Although Rachel's requested transfer to the domestic space of the kitchenware department at the end of the story similarly may seem to imply that this self is fixed in its representation, her identity continues to be defined by its relationship to consumer goods. In making Rachel's difference a source of pride, however, the text counters the pathologizing essentialism of nativist thought. In "The Girl Who Went Right," clothing —in the ease of its production and reproduction—may point to the flimsiness of the separations between classes and ethno-racial groups, but the story never provides Rachel with the means to fashion an alternative to such dichotomies. As a shopgirl whose position selling lingerie eroticizes and commodifies her difference, especially as she is called upon to model for customers, Rachel exemplifies how women are used to sell products, always in danger of becoming objects of exchange, even in their seemingly active roles as consumers and sellers.[27] Thus, in its use of sartorial imagery, "The Girl Who Went Right" does not imagine, as Bourne does, a dynamic weaving together of ethnic identities into a novel fabric.

In contrast to Rachel, however, Ferber's other fictional saleswomen fare better in exerting agency in order to redefine the terms of identity. As full-fledged entrepreneurs and members of the managerial class, Emma McChesney and Fanny Brandeis do not just sell fashion, they also have a hand in shaping the contours of femininity. Though they mostly overlook the issue of ethnic identity, the Emma McChesney stories focus on the ways that ideologies of gender and class are both upheld and subverted in the fashion industry. In *Fanny Herself*, Ferber echoes many of the same themes of her earlier magazine series, but the 1917 novel devotes considerable time to addressing how its heroine's self-fashionings are dependent on ethnicity as well as class and gender. As a clothes buyer for a mail-order concern, Fanny Brandeis, promotes fashions that transcend class and gender differences, ultimately rejecting her business career to follow her true passion for art. In the following section, I explore how *Fanny Herself* combines Kallen's artistic metaphor of the symphony and Bourne's sartorial imagery to offer a model of cultural pluralism that counters both nativist thought and the dilution of ethnic specificity through the melting pot.

Fanny Herself *and the Fashioning of Transnational Identity*

Although it is a passing novel, *Fanny Herself*, like "The Girl Who Went Right," does not espouse passing as a means of dealing with one's ethnic or racial difference, but rather employs the trope as a critique of melting pot ideology. As Fanny comes to regret her decision to pass, the novel advocates race pride, and, in reclaiming her ethnic heritage, Fanny subsequently moves toward embracing a pluralist ideal. Growing up in the Midwestern town of Winnebago, Wisconsin, where the Brandeises are one of the few Jewish families and where her mother, Molly, supports the family by operating a dry-goods store, Brandeis' Bazaar, Fanny initially believes that her Jewish difference is a "handicap." Learning from Molly's example, Fanny develops the business acumen that provides her with a means of independence following the deaths of her parents. Feeling confined by small-town life, Fanny sets out for the big city of Chicago in search of new opportunities. There, finding both her Jewishness and her gender to be obstacles in her pursuit of a business career, she hides her ethnic background in order to procure a job at a mail order clothing company. At the end of the novel, Fanny becomes another "girl who went right," reclaiming her ethnic roots and making the decision to pursue art rather than business. The text also intimates that the adamantly self-reliant Fanny will finally settle down, since the story ends with a romantic reunion between her and her childhood acquaintance, the Jewish writer Clarence Heyl. Negotiating between what Werner Sollors has termed "consent" and "descent," Fanny, in choosing to identify as Jewish (rather than having this difference imposed upon her), transforms her difference into an "asset" rather than a handicap.[28]

Like "The Girl Who Went Right," in which the Jewishness of the protagonist goes unnamed, *Fanny Herself* maintains ambiguity about what Jewishness is, even as it clearly labels Fanny Brandeis a Jew. The influence of pluralist theories on Ferber is evident in *Fanny Herself*, especially as the protagonist participates in fairly heavy-handed didactic debates early in the novel about how to define her Jewish identity if it cannot be understood as either a race or a religion. Rather than eliding her Jewishness or making it the dominant feature of her identity, Fanny ultimately effects a metaphorical interweaving that is highly suggestive of Bourne's notion of transnationality. Fanny's refashioning of her identity in pluralistic terms resonates with many of Ferber's statements about her own Jewish allegiances in her autobiography, *A Peculiar Treasure*. Taken from Exodus 19:5 ("Now therefore, if ye will obey my voice indeed, and keep my covenant, then ye shall be a peculiar treasure unto me above all people"), the memoir's title portrays Jewish identity as an asset. The autobiography becomes a forum for Ferber to express pride in her Jewish identity, believing herself "especially privileged" to be a Jew. Contrary to the claims of some critics, Ferber did not erase Jewishness from her life or her fiction; instead, she wove together her Jewish and American identities in such a way that her ability to do so came to stand in for a national ideal. A decade before it would become commonplace for Jewish-American writers such as Norman Mailer and Saul Bellow to construct the Jew as national allegory, Ferber declared the United States "to be the Jew among the nations."[29] Ferber's use of a passing narrative in *Fanny Herself* similarly counters the notion that Jews erased their ethnic specificity and became white through their assimilation into American society. Instead, Ferber, like Kallen and Bourne, proposes that Jews redefined what it meant to be American in the process of inserting themselves into a national narrative. In setting her novel in the apparel industry, Ferber uses fashion as a material metaphor to challenge essentialist notions of immutable identity; fashion becomes a means to suggest that different versions of the self can be woven together to create new and dynamic entities, thus depicting both individual and national identity as plural and dynamic, rather than singular and static.

Like Rachel Wiletzky's, Fanny's "difference" is not so easily defined; it is at once difference from the majority and difference from one's own ethnic group that establishes Ferber's women as figures of in-betweenness. Furthermore, it becomes difficult to separate Fanny's Jewish difference from her gender difference, especially as they are both impediments to her business career. Beginning with descriptions of Fanny's mother, Molly, the differences and contradictions embodied by both Brandeis women are represented through dress. Unlike the protagonist of "The Girl Who Went Right," however, the female characters are not simply imitating fashion's dictates, but instead setting the trends:

She knew when to be old-fashioned, did Mrs. Brandeis, and when to be modern. She had worn the first short walking skirt in Winnebago. It cleared the ground in a day before germs were discovered, when women's skirts trailed and flounced behind them in a cloud of dust. One of her scandalized neighbors . . . had taken her aside to tell her that no decent woman would dress that way.

"Next year," said Mrs. Brandeis, "when you are wearing one, I'll remind you of that." And she did, too. She had worn shirtwaists with a broad "Gibson" shoulder tuck, when other Winnebago women were still encased in linings and bodices. (3)

Drawing on the rhetoric of dress reform with its emphasis on health and rationality, this passage describes Molly's flair for the practical and the functional as an initial step toward more modern dress. Embodying contradictions between the old-fashioned and the modern, Molly's style of dress reflects the sartorial changes of the turn of the century, especially with its reference to the Gibson look. Despite her curvaceous silhouette, the Gibson Girl, based on the sketches by illustrator Charles Dana Gibson, was notable for her tailored style, emphasizing a bustle rather than a long train. She came to represent the new, more independent American woman, albeit one still limited in this independence.[30]

As the above passage suggests, Molly Brandeis and, by extension, her daughter are marked by those around them as different, indecent even, due to their failure to adhere to familial, domestic, and gender conventions. Their inability to conform to Winnebago society is compounded by their racial or ethnic difference. In contrast to Ferber's own family, which was forced to move their dry-goods store from Ottumwa, Iowa, to Appleton, Wisconsin, due to anti-Semitism, the Brandeises do not suffer from severe social ostracism, but they are portrayed as exotic others, as evidenced by references to the store as an "Oriental bazaar" (3) and Fanny as a "little Oriental" (25). The peculiarity of Molly's business career is established in relation to her ethnic difference, but in a somewhat unusual way, as it turns out that Molly's work distinguishes her both from gentiles and from the rest of Winnebago Jewry. Middle-class and highly assimilated, the Jews of Winnebago "were of a type to be found in every small town; prosperous, conservative, constructive citizens, clannish . . . mingling socially with their Gentile neighbors, living well, spending their money freely, taking a vast pride in the education of their children." To these upwardly mobile small-town residents, "Molly Brandeis, a Jewess, setting out to earn her living in business like a man . . . was a thing to stir

Congregation Emanu-el to its depths. Jewish women, they would tell you, did not work thus. Their husbands worked for them, or their sons, or their brothers" (11). Molly's presence is threatening to the Jewish community as they attempt to assimilate by conforming to bourgeois norms (for, as we know from "The Girl Who Went Right," lower-class Jewish women certainly did work). Her non-conformist spirit, exemplified by her attitude toward dress, dominates the novel in the legacy she bestows upon her daughter, despite the fact that Fanny, like Rachel Wiletzky, temporarily attempts to obscure her ethnic roots by adhering to the mentality of the melting pot.

Gender and ethnic difference are linked in the text's descriptions of Fanny, as with her mother. Fanny is a paradoxical figure, a "strange mixture," for instance, of "tomboy and bookworm" (26). Fanny attributes her difference in part to the fact that her mother works "like a man, in a store" and also to her Jewishness, for she is one of only two girls in her school to stay home on the Jewish holidays. While she acknowledges that these two factors set her apart, the text goes on to state that they did "not constitute the real difference. . . . The real difference was temperamental, or emotional, or dramatic, or histrionic, or all four" (24). This description begins by echoing pseudoscientific claims about a distinct Jewish temperament, but it quickly translates temperamental difference into performativity. Like Rachel Wiletzky's, Fanny's Jewishness is associated with her dramatic tendencies. In this sentence, the use of the conjunction "or" appears to establish alternatives, while the final phrase, "all four," undermines this separation of terms to suggest that they are all possible at once—which is not that surprising given that there is a fine line between the adjectives "temperamental," "emotional," "dramatic," and "histrionic."

Written during a time when scientific notions of a Jewish race were being disseminated and simultaneously disproved, the novel wavers between a biological definition of Jewish identity and an acknowledgement of racial difference as historically and socially constructed. Fanny, for example, is described as "not what is known as the Jewish type" (91). The reference to a "Jewish type" suggests a classification based on physiognomy, even as Fanny defies such a categorization. In referring to "Jewish types," the novel draws on Maurice Fishberg's 1911 book *The Jews: A Study of Race and Environment*. Defining Jewish identity in terms of the soul rather than the body, Fishberg countered claims that Jews were biologically predisposed to illnesses of the nervous system such as hysteria; rather than refute the Jewish propensity toward mental disease, he argues that it is environmental, due, for example, to urban living and centuries of persecution. Fishberg contends that there is no "eternal Hebrew" beneath the cloak, but that the cloak itself is responsible for creating differences (an argument echoed in Gilman's hypothesis about sex distinction). The characterization of a "Jewish type" is "less than skin deep," wrote Fishberg. "Primarily it depends on . . . dress and deportment." Fishberg noted that if Jews were to "don the dress of [their] neighbors, the change might be magical. . . . The 'Jewishness' disappears together with the dress."[31]

In keeping with Fishberg's theories, dress becomes a focal point in the Jew's elision of difference in *Fanny Herself*. Like "The Girl Who Went Right," the novel complicates the binary between authenticity and imitation not only through representations of Jewish identity, but also through images of dress. Fanny's ability to pass for a gentile—in part due to her looks—is enhanced by her facility with clothes. Even in their provincial Midwestern town, Fanny "managed, somehow, to look miraculously well-dressed," as she adapted the material and styles her mother brought home from her buying trips (91). Fanny applies this skill at adaptation when she refashions herself after her mother's death, traveling to Chicago to take a position as a buyer at Haynes-Cooper mail order company. In this pivotal moment, Fanny expresses a familiar belief in the American dream; she resolves to "make something of herself," vowing to discard "race, religion, training" and "natural impulses" "if they stood in her away" (107). When Fanny does do away with her background, however, it is to compensate for being a woman in a man's world. Embarking on her career, she presents an identity devoid of ethnic particularity in order to overcome the "handicap" of her gender, which, to her, is more difficult to occlude. Perhaps her Jewishness is easily shed because she does not see it as essential to her identity. This notion is supported by the fact that the two versions of Fanny are represented through dress. As Fanny prepares to leave Winnebago, an article of clothing once again functions symbolically, as the last remaining link to her past. Coming across her mother's canning apron, she flings the article of clothing into the furnace and watches as it "stiffened, writhed, crumpled, sank, lay a blackened heap, dissolved. The fire bed glowed red and purple as before, except for a dark spot in its heart" (111). The remaining "dark spot in its heart" foreshadows Fanny's eventual return to her roots, suggesting that her identity, though constituted by materiality, cannot be completely dissolved. Through the image of the apron (interestingly, a symbol of both domestic femininity and working womanhood), *Fanny Herself* cautions against sundering familial ties; instead, as if from the ashes of her mother's garment, Fanny eventually forges a self that, while new, pays tribute to her ancestral legacy.

In this way, the text repeatedly hints at Fanny's inability to escape her past. Extending the analogy to clothes, Ferber's narrator reflects on Fanny's reinvention as a sartorial transformation: "How could she think it possible to shed her past life, like a garment? . . . She might don a new cloak to cover the old dress beneath, but the old would always be there, its folds peeping out here and there, its outlines plainly to be seen" (130). In this description, seemingly inconsistent clothing metaphors complicate the notion of essential identity. In its reference to the "new cloak," the passage seems to echo Andree's statement that all the Jew "adopts is but a cloak," yet also notable is the reference to the "old dress" beneath. Thus, the passage presents a philosophy more akin to Fishberg's argument, which views difference itself as a function of clothes. The prediction that Fanny's "old dress" will continue to peep out behind the new garment indicates that her imitation is not seamless. Like the rip in Rachel's shirt-waist in "The Girl Who Went Right," this description speaks to the ambivalence of her racial mimicry.

Where nativists saw biological difference disguised by outer garments, Ferber's novel portrays both the old and new selves in terms of dress. And if these selves are represented in material terms, they have the potential to be woven together, as in Bourne's analogy. Fanny's talent for weaving together supposedly mismatched elements is initially represented in the clothing lines she creates. Ironically, her skill at manufacturing such hybrid creations comes to the fore just as she makes the decision to discard her Jewish identity. In a transition appropriate for someone who has undergone a rebirth, she begins work as a buyer for infants' wear. Noting that the company fails to understand the desires of working-class and immigrant mothers, Fanny vows to give female customers "silver-spoon models at pewter prices" (148). Fanny's approach to sales gives cause to the Veblenian fear of mass-produced goods; it demonstrates how consumption has the potential to disrupt firmly entrenched divisions between classes as well as among ethnic groups.

Fanny employs similar tactics when she moves up in the ranks to women's wear. Hiring the haute-couture designer Camille (possibly based on Chanel) to design a line of inexpensive dresses aimed at the average middle-class woman, Fanny campaigns for styles that erode socio-economic barriers and combine masculine and feminine elements. In pitching her concept of the Camille-designed dress to the firm, Fanny makes the point that it is not only upper-class women who are privy to "what's being worn on Fifth avenue" (226), insisting on the democratizing promise of dress and consumerism. In addition to destabilizing class boundaries, the designs Fanny promotes also redefine—but do not outright reject—femininity. Fanny aims to bring her female customers the "plain, good looking little blue serge dress with a white collar and some tailored buttons,"

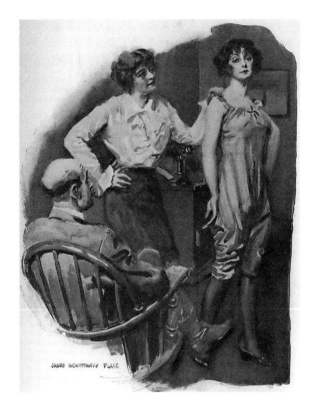

Figure 9.2 James Montgomery Flagg, "'No man will ever appreciate the fine points of this little garment, but the women—!'" Illustration in Edna Ferber's *Roast Beef, Medium: The Business Adventures of Emma McChesney* (Frederick A. Stokes Company, 1913). Rare Book and Manuscript Library, University of Pennsylvania.

a style in opposition to the accentuated femininity of the Victorian corset. At the same time, in describing Camille's innovations, Fanny notes that the renowned designer "introduced the slouch, revived the hoop, [and] discovered the sunset chiffon" (227), thus infusing her fashions with elements of a reconstructed femininity.[32]

Even as Fanny sees the potential to erode constructed boundaries of class and gender in the clothes she sells, she continues to adhere to an ideal of realness in her own wardrobe. She does not yet apply the strategy of hybridity to her Jewish and American identities, as indicated in the descriptions of her dress as she rises in the world of business. Her "blouses showed *real* Cluny ... and her hats were nothing but line"; her "sleeve flowed from arm-pit to thumb-bone without a ripple"; and the cost of her clothes was commensurate with their look (228). This depiction challenges the prediction that Fanny's "old dress" would disrupt the seamlessness of her imitation. However, Fanny's outward perfection does not necessarily correlate with her inner feeling, since she suffers from a malaise she cannot name. As the second half of the novel progresses, Fanny's loneliness is attributed to the fact that she has cut off a part of herself, and she is increasingly drawn to those she calls "my people" (261), albeit through interclass identifications. Fanny is reminded of the lost dimension of her self through her identification with women who are beneath her in the social hierarchy, and her compassion for other working women is based largely on ethnic solidarity. For example, Fanny takes a special interest in one of her factory workers, a "rather different looking" Jewish girl with "exquisite coloring, a discontented expression, and a blouse that's too low in the neck." As another character notes, this "might be a description of Fanny Brandeis, barring the blouse" (225). This comment serves as a reminder that only material conditions separate Fanny from the female factory worker, who ends up on the streets when she cannot support herself on her seven-dollar-a-week wage. Fanny's identification leads her to protest such low wages, the first indication that her social consciousness will prevail over her desire for financial status. At the same time that Fanny is drawn empathetically to the immigrant factory workers in her employ, a creative impulse propels her toward the ghetto, where she finds solace in sketching its residents and, through those sketches, begins to contemplate an alternative career path.

By the novel's end, Fanny applies the technique of combining contradictory elements to her own life. As Fanny moves toward reclaiming her Jewish identity, the novel unfolds with a romantic resolution in which she acknowledges her love for her childhood friend, Clarence Heyl, who is described as a distinct Jewish type. Fanny's "homecoming" is figured as a return to *nature*; she travels to Colorado in search of Clarence, finding herself revitalized by the mountain air, which makes her "whole again" (311). But the ending is slightly more complex than this. Although Fanny worries that she and Clarence are an incongruous pair, she allows him to persuade her that their lack of compatibility is a boon. His defense of their union echoes the ideology of cultural pluralism in which differences, rather than clashing, can combine to create a richer whole. In attempting to arrive at a strategic reconciliation of their differences, the couple decides to live simultaneously in the country and the city, traveling between Clarence's home in the mountains of Colorado and Fanny's comfort zone, the urban centers of Chicago and New York. Finally, another significant change marks the novel's denouement. Fanny decides to quit her job in order to indulge her artistic inclinations, embarking on a new career as a newspaper cartoonist. In her sketches, such as one of a Jewish garment worker leading a suffrage parade, Fanny's work takes a more explicitly political bent, but much like her career in the fashion industry, it continues to testify to the shifting ideologies of the time, depicting a nation in which women, immigrants, and the working class were contributing their voices. Thus Fanny's shift in occupation is not described in terms of one identity replacing another; instead it is a merging of identities. Observing the cartoonist at work, the narrator states: "Fanny Brandeis, the artist, and Fanny Brandeis, the salesman, combined shrewdly to omit no telling detail" (257).

In one of the few critical analyses of Ferber's fiction, June Sochen identifies *Fanny Herself* as a transitional work in the author's career. She argues that the autobiographical novel was an "exorcism" of Ferber's Jewish identity, freeing her to focus on heroines who were ethnically and religiously unidentified and allowing her to refashion herself as an American writer.[33] Ferber does indeed broaden her repertoire after *Fanny Herself*, producing a series of blockbuster regional novels—including *So Big*, *Show Boat*, *Cimarron*, *Saratoga Trunk*, and *Giant*—with non-Jewish heroines. Yet, in documenting a diverse, multiethnic panorama of the nation, these novels expose a partially hidden history of interracialism in order to underscore how cultural mixing is fundamental to American identity. Ferber's work thus continued to promote the pluralistic ethos she first explored through her Jewish heroine in *Fanny Herself*. Fanny Brandeis, it turns out, is not so much a ghost of Ferber's past as a prototype for her heroine of the future; she provides a model for the spirited, self-reliant, and border-crossing working women who populate the writer's fictional universe. Ferber's later novels may forego the fashion industry setting for a more expansive terrain of American life, but her protagonists continue to exhibit impeccable taste in clothes and, more importantly, an awareness of how dress can be enlisted strategically to construct and reconstruct their identities.

In the earliest stages of her career, Ferber located fashion as a site that allows us to re-examine the terms of modernity through the lens of femininity. The images of fashion in her fiction elucidate the modern concept of a plural self in which differences can coexist rather than collide. The ambivalences engendered by fashion continue to plague feminist theorists today. While dress can be potentially liberating for women, especially in the way it draws attention to the construction of femininity, some feminist scholars view fashion as a form of capitalist and patriarchal oppression because they perceive of the fashion and beauty industries as male-dominated institutions, as Naomi Wolf famously argued in *The Beauty Myth*. Ferber's stories, however, present a counter-narrative, one that endorses the findings of historians such as Valerie Steele and Kathy Peiss who have emphasized the role that women (and, for Peiss, specifically ethnic women) have played in these industries.[34] Chronicling female professionalization in the early twentieth century, Ferber's fiction portrays women as both embodiments and agents of the modern. Her protagonists resist the conformity typically associated with fashion for the agency of refashioning their identities. Along with the work of contemporaries such as Yezierska and Fauset, Ferber's writing further encourages a rethinking of feminist analyses of fashion by partaking in the discourse of cultural pluralism. She challenges the nativist notion that ethnic others would corrupt "the fabric of our race," promoting instead a transnational ideal in which the fabric of the nation is strengthened and enriched through the interweaving of differences. In the figure of Fanny Brandeis, Ferber created a heroine who innovates design to redefine the ways that gender, race, ethnicity, and class were constructed by the dominant culture and, in the process, invested fashion with new meanings that made it much "more than a garment."

Notes

1. Henry Cabot Lodge, "The Restriction of Immigration," in *Speeches and Addresses, 1884–1909* (Boston and New York: Houghton Mifflin Company, 1909), 245–66.

2. Madison Grant, *The Passing of the Great Race* (New York: Charles Scribner's Sons, 1916), 81.

3. Cited in Sander Gilman, *The Jew's Body* (New York and London: Routledge, 1991), 76.

4. E. A. Ross, *The Old World In the New* (New York: The Century Company, 1914), 285–86.

5. Israel Zangwill, *The Melting-Pot* [1909] (New York: Macmillan, 1920), 33–34.

6. For more on Ford's melting pot ceremony, see Lawrence W. Levine, *The Opening of the American Mind: Canons, Culture, and History* (Boston: Beacon Press, 1996), chapter 6.

7. Horace Kallen, "Democracy versus the Melting-Pot," in *A Norton Anthology of Jewish American Literature* (New York: W.W. Norton, 2001), 207–17.

8. Randolph Bourne, "Trans-National America," in *War and the Intellectuals* (New York: Harper & Row, 1964), 107–23.

9. Thorstein Veblen, *The Theory of the Leisure Class* (New York: Dover, 1994), 106.

10. Charlotte Perkins Gilman, *The Dress of Women,* ed. Michael R. Hill and Mary Jo Deegan (Westport, CT: Greenwood Press, 2002), 39, 34.

11. See Valerie Steele, "Chanel in Context," in *Chic Thrills: A Fashion Reader,* ed. Elizabeth Wilson and Julie Ash (Berkeley: University of California Press, 1992), 118–26. Additional background on Chanel can be found in Edmonde Charles-Roux, *Chanel and Her World* (New York: Vendome Press, 1981); and Janet Wallach, *Chanel: Her Style and Her Life* (New York: Doubleday, 1998).

12. Recent scholarship that draws on fashion theory has begun to take note of these intersections. See, for example, Alys Eve Weinbaum et al., ed., *The Mod-*

ern Girl Around the World: Consumption, Modernity, and Globalization (Durham, NC: Duke University Press, 2008); and Emma Tarlo, *Visibly Muslim: Fashion, Politics, Faith* (New York: Berg, 2010).

13. For further discussion of Jewish immigrant women workers in the garment industry, see Nancy L. Green, *Ready-to-Wear and Ready-to-Work: A Century of Industry and Immigrants in Paris and New York* (Durham, NC: Duke University Press, 1997); Elizabeth Ewen, *Immigrant Women in the Land of Dollars: Life and Culture on the Lower East Side, 1890–1925* (New York: Monthly Review Press, 1985); and Barbara Schreier, *Becoming American Women: Clothing and Jewish Immigrant Experience, 1880–1920* (Chicago: Chicago Historical Society, 1994).

14. For literary criticism on images of fashion in Yezierska and Fauset, see Christopher Okonkwo, "Of Repression, Assertion, and the Speakerly Dress: Anzia Yezierska's *Salome of the Tenements,*" *MELUS* 25, no. 1 (Spring 2000), 129–45; Meredith Goldsmith, "Dressing, Passing, and Americanizing: Anzia Yezierska's Sartorial Fictions," *Studies in American Jewish Literature* 16 (1997), 34–45; Meredith Goldsmith, "'The Democracy of Beauty': Fashioning Ethnicity and Gender in the Fiction of Anzia Yezierska," *Yiddish/Modern Jewish Studies* 11, no. 3–4 (1999), 166–87; Katherine Stubbs, "Reading Material: Contextualizing Clothing in the Work of Anzia Yezierska," *MELUS* 23, no. 2 (Summer 1998), 157–72; and my own "No Slaves to Fashion: Designing Women in the Fiction of Jessie Fauset and Anzia Yezierska," in *Styling Texts: Dress and Fashion in Literature*, ed. Cynthia Kuhn and Cindy Carlson (New York: Cambria Press, 2007), 313–33.

15. Joyce Kilmer, "Business Woman Most Domestic," *New York Times* (April 4, 1915): 4.

16. See Bourne, "Trans-National America," 113–14; and "Trans-Nationalism and the Jew," in *War and the Intellectuals* (New York: Harper & Row, 1964): 124–33. Bourne also mentions in the latter essay that the term "trans-nationalism" was coined by a Jewish classmate.

17. Kallen, "Democracy versus the Melting-Pot," 213.

18. Edna Ferber, *A Peculiar Treasure* (New York: Doubleday, 1939), 6. Biographical background on Ferber can also be found in Julie Goldsmith Gilbert, *Ferber: A Biography* (New York: Doubleday, 1978); Carolyn Heilbrun, "Edna Ferber," in *Notable American Women: The Modern Period*, ed. Barbara Sicherman and Carol Hurd Green (Cambridge, MA: Harvard University Press, 1980); Joyce Antler, *The Journey Home: Jewish Women and the American Century* (New York: Free Press, 1997), 150–72; and Marion Meade, *Bobbed Hair and Bathtub Gin: Writers Running Wild in the Twenties* (New York: Harcourt, 2004).

19. Edna Ferber, "The Girl Who Went Right," in *America and I: Short Stories By American Jewish Women Writers*, ed. Joyce Antler (Boston: Beacon Press, 1990), 66. Further references will be cited parenthetically in the text.

20. Mary Antin, *The Promised Land* [1912] (New York: Penguin, 1997), 3. Other literary examples of Jewish immigrants using similar sartorial imagery include Emma Goldman, whose labor activism began in the dressmaking trade and who described herself as casting off her prior life "like a worn-out garment" when she arrived in New York City several years after her emigration from Russia (Emma Goldman, *Living My Life*, [New York: Dover, 1970 (1931)], 3); and Abraham Cahan's eponymous protagonist in *The Rise of David Levinsky* (1917), who

establishes himself in the New World as a cloak-manufacturer and views the garment industry as a crucial stepping-stone in his Americanization.

21. Homi Bhabha, *The Location of Culture* (New York: Routledge, 1994), 89.

22. Nan Enstad, *Ladies of Labor, Girls of Adventure: Working Women, Popular Culture, and Labor Politics at the Turn of the Twentieth Century* (New York: Columbia University Press, 1999), 66.

23. Thorstein Veblen, *The Theory of the Leisure Class*, 104.

24. Tania Modleski, "Femininity as Mas(s)querade: A Feminist Approach to Mass Culture," in *High Theory/Low Culture*, ed. Colin MacCabe (New York: St. Martin's Press, 1986), 37–52.

25. See Gilman, *The Jew's Body*; and Daniel Itzkovitz, "Passing Like Me: Jewish Chameleonism and the Politics of Race," in *Passing: Identity and Interpretation in Sexuality, Race, and Religion*, ed. Maria Carla Sanchez and Linda Schlossberg (New York: New York University Press, 2001), 38–63.

26. See Susan Benson, *Counter Cultures: Saleswoman, Managers, and Customers in American Department Stores, 1890–1940* (Urbana: University of Illinois Press, 1988): 135.

27. At the same time, Rachel's position as a model allows her to operate outside the conventional heterosexual economy, suggesting what Diana Fuss calls a "homospectatorial look," since it is other women, both costumers and salesgirls, who ogle Rachel's appearance. As Fuss argues, the fashion industry "provides a socially sanctioned structure in which women are encouraged to *consume*, in voyeuristic if not vampiristic fashion, the images of other women." While the "homospectatorial look" creates an ambivalence between identification and desire, it also gets at the ambivalence of fashion itself, which operates simultaneously as a re-enforcer of hegemonic values and as a potential site for subversion. See Fuss, "Fashion and the Homospectatorial Look," in *On Fashion*, ed. Shari Benstock and Suzanne Ferris (New Brunswick, NJ: Rutgers University Press, 1994), 211.

28. Werner Sollors, *Beyond Ethnicity: Consent and Descent in American Culture* (New York: Oxford University Press, 1986); Edna Ferber, *Fanny Herself* (Urbana: University of Illinois Press, 2001 [1917]), 121. Further references to *Fanny Herself* will be cited parenthetically in the text.

29. Ferber, *Peculiar Treasure*, 9, 10. On the Jew as national allegory, see Daniel Itzkovitz, "Secret Temples," in *Jews and Other Differences*, ed. Jonathan Boyarin and Daniel Boyarin (Minneapolis: University of Minnesota Press, 1997), 177.

30. On the Gibson Girl, see, for example, Martha Banta, *Imaging American Women* (New York: Columbia University Press, 1987).

31. Maurice Fishberg, *The Jews: A Study of Race and Environment* (New York: Charles Scribner, 1911), 162–63.

32. Similar images of fashion as a symbol of hybridity appear in the writings of Anzia Yezierska. In Yezierska's 1923 novel, *Salome of the Tenements*, for example, the fashion designer protagonist, Sonya Vrunsky, makes her name by bringing seemingly antithetical elements together. Her legendary creation, "The Sonya Model," is described as "a costume, plain enough for everybody but distinctive enough to make it effective for any occasion," allowing "the wearer to have the joy of a dress that could be slipped on in a moment, and yet give the luxurious

sense of a fitted gown. A supple, clinging thing in everyday serge, veiling yet revealing the lovely curves of a woman's body" (Anzia Yezierska, *Salome of the Tenements*, [Chicago: University of Illinois Press, 1995], 169).

33. June Sochen, *Consecrate Every Day: The Public Lives of Jewish American Women, 1880–1980* (Albany: State University of New York Press, 1981), 103–105.

34. See Naomi Wolf, *The Beauty Myth: How Images of Beauty Are Used Against Women* (New York: Doubleday, 1991); Valerie Steele, "Chanel in Context"; and Kathy Peiss, *Hope in a Jar: The Making of America's Beauty Culture* (New York: Henry Holt, 1998).

Rita Felski

AFTERWORD

While reading through this lucid and engaging group of essays, I was reminded anew of how much has changed in feminist studies and modernist studies over the last two decades. What once seemed outré is now acceptable, even self-evident; what once furrowed eyebrows and engendered looks of consternation is accepted with nary a murmur. When we ponder changes in thinking, our attention is often caught by breaks and ruptures, paradigm shifts, moments of conversion—iconoclasm, after all, makes for a more riveting story. And yet, we surely glean a better sense of how knowledge changes by seeing how once-eccentric ideas are absorbed, internalized, and put to work—allowing us to expend much less effort on defending such ideas and more on using, expanding, and elaborating them.

Several essays in this collection, for example, explore the modernity of women's experience in middle or late-Victorian culture without feeling the need to belabor the ways in which such experience counts as modern. What a difference from the 1980s, when "Victorian" and "modern" were widely taken as antonyms rather than synonyms and the nineteenth century was often condescended to, or even rebuked, for its retrograde realism and hidebound traditionalism. No longer bound to the experimental art of the early to mid-twentieth century, "modern" has acquired for literary critics the amplitude and reach of historical reference that it has long enjoyed elsewhere. This uncoupling of modernity from aesthetic modernism also helps explain the eclectic range of topics explored in this collection, whether Elizabeth Sheehan's treatment of purportedly conservative works of African-American art, Justine De Young's analysis of once-notorious French paintings overshadowed by the technical innovations of the Impressionist canon, Ellen Bayuk Rosenman's survey of responses to the mid-Victorian coquette, or Christina Bates's account of the social semiotics of nursing uniforms. Taken as a whole, the collection eloquently confirms that when women become central rather than peripheral to theories of modernity, our assumptions about what counts as conservative or modern, traditional or transgressive, are suddenly in flux.

While the modern looks quite different than it did two decades ago, feminist thought has also undergone some key changes. The essays in this volume embrace views on agency, culture, and politics far removed from the kinds of arguments that were in vogue when I began thinking about gender and modernity two decades ago. The absolutist tone of either/or thinking is notably absent: the frantic search for a zone of otherness untouched by patriarchal encroachments; the insistence that the masculine structures of modernity—whether linguistic or institutional—will automatically pulverize any attempt at female actualization or expression. Instead of theories of phallocentric structures and occluded female agency, the language of "negotiation" now holds sway, used or implied in the work of virtually all the contributors. The tone is set in the introduction, when Ilya Parkins and Elizabeth Sheehan argue that "fashion enables us to conceptualize modernity not as an imposition, but rather as a negotiation." In her account of the cultural meanings of British tea gowns and aesthetic dress, Kimberly Wahl comments that, "women actively negotiated the complex terrain of social roles available to them." Discussing the details of the British secondhand clothing trade, Celia Marshik writes that women "did not so much consume interwar fashion as negotiate it." And in her description of Fauset's novels and VanDerZee's photographs, Sheehan speaks of both "negotiation" and "adaptation," suggesting that clothing offered various possibilities "for adjusting the norms and practices of race and gender."

What lies behind this shift in terminology and its impact on our ideas about gender, fashion, and modernity? Adorning the title of one of Stephen Greenblatt's works, *Shakespearian Negotiations*, and furnishing one of the key terms of New Historicism, the idea of negotiation also has quite an independent genealogy in film theory, cultural studies, and reception aesthetics. As used by Greenblatt, the term has economic resonances, conveying how works of art draw on circulating social energies via various forms of appropriation, acquisition, transaction, and symbolic exchange. More generally, Greenblatt's notion of self-fashioning has affinities with this collection's focus on how women used fashion to create themselves as particular kinds of people. Indeed, the popularity of a phrase such as "negotiating gender"—which now adorns a multitude of book and essay subtitles—underscores how feminists are increasingly inclined to conceive the condition of being female or male as neither inherent and inborn nor unilaterally imposed by ideological fiat, but as painstakingly achieved through interaction between diverse—even if unequally powerful—parties. It is, in other words, a resolutely dialectical concept, insisting on the inescapability of interrelation between phenomena and gauging the gains as well as the losses of such interrelation.

In a parallel though rarely overlapping history, the concept of negotiation was seized on by film scholars and cultural studies critics in the 1980s in order to challenge deterministic accounts of mass media forms as coercing and controlling viewers. A key intervention was Christine Gledhill's oft-cited "Pleasurable Negotiations," which explicitly pitched its argument against then-current psychoanalytical and poststructuralist models of textual meaning. "The term negotiation," writes Gledhill, "implies the holding together of opposite sides in an ongoing process of give and take . . . Meaning is neither imposed, nor passively imbibed, but arises out of a struggle or negotiation between competing frames of reference, motivation, or experience."[1] Such negotiation, moreover, is not only political, but, as her title suggests, infused with a plenitude of yearnings, desires, impulses, and attachments. A shift in terminology and in method opened up new possibilities for a serious engagement with (rather than tight-lipped diagnosis of) the emotions and attachments of audiences.

This intellectual legacy—of acknowledging agency and pleasure in women's dialectical relationship to larger structures—makes negotiation a concept that is especially well suited to the discussion of fashion. As various contributors to this collection point out, fashion is both public and intimate, macro and micro, structural and phenomenological: a global, multi-headed leviathan steered by industrial and seasonal rhythms as well as often opaque market forces, but also an irreducibly personal connection to the materials that drape and adorn our bodies—a second skin, if you will, imprinted with often potent memories and personal histories, an individually customized semiotic that conveys silent yet eloquent messages about who we are or would like to become. That fashion involves both art and emotion seems an obvious point—and yet one whose implications we sometimes fail to explore in our eagerness to calibrate the precise degree to which clothing serves to subvert or sustain social hierarchies.

Here the work of Bruno Latour offers a pertinent resource for feminist engagements with fashion. First of all, there is Latour's well-known insistence on the importance of things, the coevalness and co-dependence of people and objects, which seems especially well suited to conceiving fashion as an actor that creates rather than simply reflects modernity, in the words of Parkins and Sheehan. Fashion, in this line of thought, is not a reflex or epiphenomenon of larger structures of patriarchy or capitalism;

rather it is an agent—that is, something whose presence makes a difference —as well as an intermediary that actively translates—rather than faithfully transmitting—prior social meanings. For example, in a suggestive aside on the difference between nylon and silk, Latour warns against reading such materials only as reflections of preexisting divisions between lower-class and upper-class taste, arguing that we need to attend to "the many indefi-nite material nuances between the feel, the touch, the color, the sparkling of silk and nylon" that bring new perceptions and meanings into play.[2] We miss the singularity of these differences if we treat them only as il-lustrations of a prior social scheme. Let us fully describe the objects of fashion, in other words, before hastening to explain them.

There is, I believe, also much to be learned from Latour's energetic dismantling of critique, as a mode of thinking that can only account for the motives and desires of human beings by appealing to more-or-less sophisticated models of false consciousness. Critique, in other words, arrogates to itself the authority of enlightened thought and is willing to rubber-stamp only those forms of activity that accord with its concep-tion of what counts as radical, oppositional, or subversive action. The difficulty here is two-fold: first, a failure to come to terms with modes of experience that elude such measurement and that are shoe-horned into political pigeonholes at a significant cost; second, an inattentiveness to the emotionally infused and non-rational elements of critique itself. To give fashion its due, we need to be able to ask questions other than: "is it hegemonic?" "Is it subversive?" (Questions like these allow for only a few possible answers: "yes," "no," or, inevitably, "it's both!") Such an approach surely fails to get to the heart of why fashion seduces, dazzles, enchants, endures. It looks through fashion—to meanings presumed to remain hidden to participants themselves—rather than at fashion—as ex-perience, promise, image, fantasy, expression, dream, transformation, ideal. The goal of a Latourian analysis, in other words, is to increase or bolster the reality of the phenomenon being studied rather than to diminish or deplete it.

The worry, to be sure, is that in foregoing critique we are abandoning politics. In fact, we are only abstaining from a particular style of politics, one cast in the mode of judgment, in which we draw up taxonomies of behavior by ranking their oppressive or emancipatory effects. Given that virtually any aspect of fashion can be proved to be either thoroughly radi-cal or utterly retrograde by an ingeniously minded critic, however, this may be less of a loss to knowledge than it first appears. Let us envisage a different kind of politics, one that is not about judging, but about assem-bling, not about dismantling, but about collecting and composing, not about subjugating phenomena to our preexisting categories, but about fully engaging the reality of such phenomena, especially when they elude or expand our ingrained modes of thought. The goal of such a politics, in other words, is to reckon with the chaotic multiplicity of actors, intermediaries, and attachments at work in fashion, including those we may be tempted to label anachronistic, ideological, or mystifying. It is a question of treating phenomena in all their amplitude, rather than seeing them as screens for hidden social forces.

An intriguing motif that surfaces at various points in this collection, for example, is the question of character. What is the relationship between fashion and character, between what we wear and who we are? As the essays by Rosenman, Tennant, and De Young demonstrate with verve and clarity, this topic was a recurring source of fascination and speculation in the nineteenth century. Countless pages were devoted to detailing what women's appearance revealed about their attitudes, conduct, and inner worth. The visual was yoked to the moral, and clothing taken as a revealing index of personality and standing. Of course, as these essays show, such hopes were often mistaken; clothing was by no means easily deciphered, there were frequent disjunctions between appearance and behavior, and the democratization of fashion muddied and muddled distinctions between ladies and ladies of the night, between gentlemen and parvenus. What Tennant writes about Beraud's painting holds true of fashion itself: the more closely we look at it, "the more it beguiles us . . . the more it evades a single, stable, reading."

We might conclude, then, that notions of morality and character are a bad dream from which we have now awakened, that we have shrugged off the benighted ideas of earlier epochs. Yet contemporary blogs, TV shows, and magazines are, of course, awash with commentary about clothing and its perceived links to morality and character, whether the subject is Paris Hilton or Hillary Clinton. And if we're inclined to explain such speculations as residual, retrograde sexism or evidence of hopelessly "pre-modern" rather than "post-modern" thinking, what do we make of the fact that our critical discussions of fashion are also saturated with moral and characterological assumptions? When we attribute subversive and scandalizing effects to the female coquette (Rosenman), when we admire Eileen Gray's sartorial disruption to heteronormative visual codes (Rault), we are, indisputably, drawing on moral categories, albeit ones that reverse traditional value schemes in order to prize the merits of dissidence, insouciance, and marginality. Such critical discriminations, moreover, involve judgments about attitude, self-presentation, and disposition that are intimately connected to the history of character. Contemporary criticism, especially, values a stance—ironic, detached, skeptical, parodic—that is not just a form of thought, but an orientation or disposition, a mode of self-presentation, an ethos, if you will. Indeed, the recent prominence of drag and cross-dressing motifs in feminist and queer theory underscores the extent to which we continue to project powerful ethical meanings onto clothing, even as the language of performance and theatricality has come, paradoxically, to signify a higher authenticity in marking its distance from normative gender regimes.[3]

While constraints of space prevent me from commenting on all the essays, let me mention a few that I found especially suggestive. On reading Justine De Young's account of Charles-François Marchal's two paintings and the cacophony of responses they inspired at the 1868 Paris Salon, I was struck by the author's adept circumvention of a well-worn feminist complaint about oppressive gender binaries. (The vicissitudes of translation are also relevant here, for "courtisane ou menagère," after all, does not carry the same resonance as "housewife or harlot." "Courtisane" assumes a chronological and perhaps conceptual priority in the French phrase that is absent in English, while conveying little of the harshness of the quintessentially Victorian "harlot.") De Young is less interested in classifying these paintings as coercive or subversive than in posing another kind of question: why were they so fascinating? And in tackling this question she also captivates us via her evocative description of Marchal's portraits and the multifarious readings, reactions, and parodies they engendered. The essay allows us to see, in Latourian terms, that the history of an artwork is the history of its attachments and that these attachments are contingent, diverse, and sometimes unpredictable, fanning out in many different directions. Responses to *Pénélope* and *Phryné* were varied in kind, involving disagreement and conflict even within a small cohort of male Parisian critics and commentators, as well as in form, involving a host of intellectual and emotional assumptions about gender, physiognomy, fashion, modernity, personhood. And in bringing these forgotten artworks so vividly to life, De Young implicates us, as readers and viewers, in many of the same questions.

Like De Young, Christina Bates approaches questions of gender, fashion, and modernity through their visual representation. Her album of photographs drives home how much the conventions of photography, as well as nurses' uniforms, have changed. It is inconceivable nowadays that a visual record of student nurses, or any other professional group, would tolerate such asymmetry of poses, expressions, and head heights. We have come to expect neatly serried ranks—straight-backed, straight-faced, row-by-row—not decorative bouquets of inclined female bodies. As the author writes: "graduate photographs of nurses are compelling; they bring us face-to-face with the experience of nurse training at this formative period. The students' expressions, the way they wear their uniforms, their gestures, and their props form a discourse about nursing culture in late-Victorian society." Bates's essay is illuminating and informative about how nursing uniforms changed over time while negotiating telling divisions of gender and class. The professionalizing of nursing demanded a uniform that would differentiate its wearers from an earlier tradition of often ad hoc, untrained, lower-class care, while also signaling a distance from the more frivolous elements of fashion. Uniforms encouraged a new sense of professional pride, authority, and expertise among the young women who wore them, marking differences of background, education, and aspiration. At the same time, pink dresses, aprons, and puffy caps also bespoke a restrained and refined femininity, separating nurses from the male doctors they served and cementing the view that tending to the sick was a naturally female occupation. Through her careful reading of bodices and bows, patched aprons and puffed sleeves, Bates's essay opens a window into a long-lost way of life, and into the power of clothes to shape the desires and identities of those who wear them.

Elizabeth Sheehan's essay overlaps with Bates in its interest in women's use of clothing to connote dignity, authority, and respectability, while underscoring the ways in which the burdens and pleasures of appearing were shaped by race. Reassessing photographic and literary work that has often been seen as apolitical, smug, or aesthetically timid, it elucidates the importance of fashion in VanDerZee's photography and Fauset's fiction as a means of self-making within a larger cultural formation of African-American modernity. (There are interesting connections here to Lori Harrison-Kahan's exploration of the links between the garment industry and contested notions of American ethnicity and transnational identity.) Clothing could speak volumes about taste and character, style and status, ambitions and aspirations, and the multifarious connections and tensions between personhood and larger forms of racial, ethnic, or national belonging. It has, in other ways, indisputable political overtones of a kind that we will fail to see if we miss fashion's intimate entanglement with romance and dreams, fantasy, and hope. Fashion inevitably falls short if measured by criteria of radical critique or revolutionary transformation, but it does offer, in Sheehan's words, "new configurations and possibilities within the sphere of the everyday."

In his recent book, *Fashion: A Philosophy*, Lars Svendsen concludes his survey of writing on fashion by denying it any deeper significance. The only truths it conveys, he suggests, are the omnipresent postmodern clichés that it also helps to actualize: "that we cultivate surfaces, that we live in an increasingly fictionalized reality, that the constancy of our identities is steadily declining."[4] Fashion, in this line of thought, is a code word for the triumph of style over substance, the worship of novelty for novelty's sake, the replacement of politics by aesthetics, the emptying out of personhood via its reduction to a performance or a brand. What this collection demonstrates, by contrast, is a dissenting view: one that sees style as substance, that refuses the antithesis of mode and meaning, that situates fashion in the heterogeneous life worlds, attachments, emotions, and aspirations of its users. Fashion, in other words, is not mere surface, superfice, or simulation, but a "lived cultural construct" (Parkins and Sheehan) that unmakes and also remakes gender, character, and personhood in modernity.

Notes

1. Christine Gledhill, "Pleasurable Negotiations," in *Female Spectators: Looking at Film and Television*, ed. E. Deidre Pribram (London: Verso, 1988).

2. Bruno Latour, *Reassembling The Social* (Oxford: Oxford University Press, 2005), 40.

3. See Amanda Anderson, *The Way We Argue Now: A Study in the Cultures of Theory* (Princeton: Princeton University, 2006).

4. Lars Svendsen, *Fashion: A Philosophy* (London: Reaktion, 2006), 157.

Contributors

CHRISTINA BATES is the curator for Ontario History at the Canadian Museum of Civilization. She curated the 2005–06 major exhibition, "A Caring Profession: Centuries of Nursing in Canada" and is co-editor of *On All Frontiers: Four Centuries of Canadian Nursing* (2005). Her special interest is the history of dress and culture.

JUSTINE DE YOUNG teaches art history, theory, and prose writing as part of the faculty of the Harvard College Writing Program. Her research interests revolve around the intersection of modernism and fashion in eighteenth and nineteenth-century art, literature, and visual culture. She received her PhD in art history from Northwestern University.

RITA FELSKI is William R. Kenan, Jr., Professor of English at the University of Virginia and editor of *New Literary History*. She is the author of *Beyond Feminist Aesthetics* (1989), *The Gender of Modernity* (1995), *Doing Time: Feminist Theory and Postmodern Culture* (2000), *Literature after Feminism* (2003), and *Uses of Literature* (2008), and editor of *Rethinking Tragedy* (2008).

LORI HARRISON-KAHAN currently teaches in the English Department at Boston College and has previously taught at Connecticut College, Harvard University, and the University of Pennsylvania. She is the author of *The White Negress: Literature, Minstrelsy, and the Black-Jewish Imaginary* (2011). Her essays have appeared in *Cinema Journal, Legacy, MELUS, Modern Fiction Studies, Modern Language Studies, Tulsa Studies in Women's Literature*, and in the anthology *Styling Texts: Dress and Fashion in Literature*.

CELIA MARSHIK is Associate Professor of English and affiliate faculty with Comparative Literature and Cultural Studies and Women's and Gender Studies at SUNY Stony Brook. Her book *British Modernism and Censorship* was published by Cambridge in 2006. Her current project, "Wearing Modernity," focuses on four types of garments that illuminate fashion's cultural codes in the 1920s and 1930s. An article from this project is forthcoming in *Modernism/modernity*.

ILYA PARKINS is Assistant Professor and Coordinator of Gender and Women's Studies at the University of British Columbia Okanagan. She holds a PhD in Social and Political Thought from York University. Her essays on fashion, feminist theory, and modernity have appeared in *Time and Society, Women's Studies, Australian Feminist Studies, Transformations*, and *Tessera*. Her current research examines the status of women and time in the life writing of three early twentieth-century French fashion designers.

JASMINE RAULT is an Assistant Professor of Women's Studies at McMaster University. Her research is on early twentieth-century visual culture, interior design, architecture, sexuality, and gender. Recent essays can be found in *Fashion and Interior Design: Embodied Practices* (2009) and *Archives of American Art Journal* (2009). She is the author of *Eileen Gray and the Design of Sapphic Modernity* (2011).

ELLEN BAYUK ROSENMAN is a Provost's Distinguished Service Professor in the English Department and a faculty affiliate of the Gender and Women's Studies Department at the University of Kentucky. She is the author of *Unauthorized Pleasures: Accounts of Victorian Erotic Experience* and co-editor with Professor Claudia Klaver of *Other Mothers: Beyond the Maternal Ideal.* She is at work on a book manuscript about penny dreadful and the social imaginaries of the Victorian working classes. She is also the editor of the *Victorians Institute Journal.*

ELIZABETH M. SHEEHAN is an Assistant Professor of English and Women's Studies affiliate at Ithaca College. Her teaching and research interests include transatlantic modernism, gender, and visual and material culture, and she has recently published an essay on avant-garde dress design of the Bloomsbury Group. She is completing a book manuscript on fashion and Anglo-American literary modernism.

KARA TENNANT completed her doctoral research at Cardiff University in 2010. Her thesis, entitled "'Graceful Expression and Useful Purpose': Mid-Victorian Fashionable Femininity," examines fashionable representations of women in the mid-Victorian period. While undertaking this work, she taught in the undergraduate program at Cardiff University for four years. She has contributed regularly to conferences in the UK, the US, and Canada. She is co-editor of a collection of essays entitled *Signs, Symbols, and Words* (2007), available online through Cardiff University's Humanities Research Institute. Her research interests include the cultural history of fashion from the late eighteenth to the early twentieth century, Victorian travel writing, and the ladies' periodical.

KIMBERLY WAHL is an Assistant Professor in the School of Fashion at Ryerson University. She holds a PhD in Art History from Queen's University in Kingston, Ontario, Canada, where her dissertation focused on dress reform in the context of British visual culture and Aestheticism. Her current research examines the relationship between fashion and feminism, historically as well as in contemporary visual culture.

Index

LIBRARY OF CONGRESS CATALOGING-IN-PUBLICATION DATA

Cultures of femininity in modern fashion / Ilya Parkins and Elizabeth M. Sheehan, editors.

    p. cm. — (Becoming modern: new nineteenth-century studies)

    Includes bibliographical references and index.

    ISBN 978-1-61168-001-0 (cloth : alk. paper) — ISBN 978-1-61168-002-7 (pbk. : alk. paper)

1. Women's clothing—Social aspects.   2. Clothing and dress—Social aspects.   3. Fashion—Social aspects.

4. Feminism—Social aspects.   I. Parkins, Ilya.   II. Sheehan, Elizabeth M.

    GT1720.C85 2011

    391'.2—DC22   2011007983